THE

Unde
and **ing myofascial**
trigger points

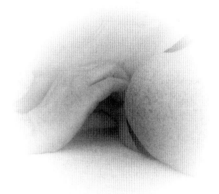

For Elsevier:

Senior Commissioning Editor: Sarena Wolfaard
Associate Editor: Claire Wilson
Project Manager: Joannah Duncan
Senior Designer: George Ajayi
Illustration Manager: Bruce Hogarth
Illustrators: Barking Dog Studios, Graeme Chambers

A MASSAGE THERAPIST'S GUIDE TO

Understanding, locating and treating myofascial trigger points

 With accompanying DVD

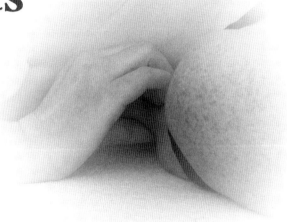

Leon Chaitow ND DO

Registered Osteopathic Practitioner and Honorary Fellow,
University of Westminster, London, UK

Sandy Fritz BS MS

Director, Health Enrichment Center,
School of Therapeutic Massage, Lapeer, MI, USA

Foreword by
Robert K. King

Illustrations by
Graeme Chambers BA(Hons)
Medical Artist

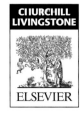

CHURCHILL
LIVINGSTONE

ELSEVIER

EDINBURGH LONDON NEW YORK OXFORD PHILADELPHIA ST LOUIS SYDNEY TORONTO 2006

CHURCHILL LIVINGSTONE
ELSEVIER

© 2006, Elsevier Ltd. All rights reserved.

The right of Leon Chaitow and Sandy Fritz to be identified as authors of this work has been asserted by them in accordance with the Copyright, Designs and Patents Act 1988

No part of this publication may be reproduced, stored in a retrieval system, or transmitted in any form or by any means, electronic, mechanical, photocopying, recording or otherwise, without either the prior permission of the Publishers. Permissions may be sought directly from Elsevier's Health Sciences Rights Department, 1600 John F Kennedy Boulevard, Suite 1800, Philadelphia, PA 19103-2899, USA: phone: (+1) 215 239 3804, fax: (+1) 215 239 3805, e-mail: healthpermissions@elsevier.com. You may also complete your request on-line via the Elsevier homepage (http://www.elsevier.com), by selecting 'Support and contact' and then 'Copyright and Permission'.

First published 2006
Reprinted 2007

ISBN 0443 10200 7
ISBN-13 978 0 443 10200 4

British Library Cataloguing in Publication Data
A catalogue record for this book is available from the British Library

Library of Congress Cataloging in Publication Data
A catalog record for this book is available from the Library of Congress

Notice
Neither the Publisher nor the Author assume any responsibility for any loss or injury and/or damage to persons or property arising out of or related to any use of the material contained in this book. It is the responsibility of the treating practitioner, relying on independent expertise and knowledge of the patient, to determine the best treatment and method of application for the patient.

The Publisher

Working together to grow
libraries in developing countries

www.elsevier.com | www.bookaid.org | www.sabre.org

ELSEVIER   BOOK AID   Sabre Foundation
             International

ELSEVIER
your source for books,
journals and multimedia
in the health sciences
www.elsevierhealth.com

Printed in China

The
publisher's
policy is to use
**paper manufactured
from sustainable forests**

Contents

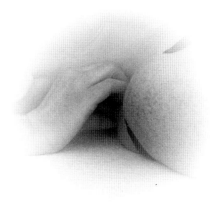

The CD-ROM accompanying this text includes video sequences of all the techniques indicated in the text by the icon. To look at the video for a given technique, click on the relevant icon in the contents list on the CD-ROM. The CD-ROM is designed to be used in conjunction with the text and not as a stand-alone product.

Foreword

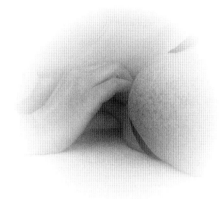

Some 20 years ago, while browsing through a British alternative health journal, I first stumbled across Leon Chaitow's essay entitled 'Whole Body May Be Trigger Point'. The article succinctly asserted what I intuitively knew: that the entire surface, indeed the total landscape of the body, was potentially an area, however minute, of a nasty form of soft tissue dysfunction that possessed pain-generating characteristics.

Since the entire encasement of our physical structure is a potential source of this peculiar irritating pain that, when provoked, stimulates noxious impulses in predictable ways, new and highly efficacious manual protocols are called for.

I am, therefore, honored to write the foreword to this vital and long overdue work. *A Massage Therapist's Guide to Understanding, Locating and Treating Myofascial Trigger Points* by Leon Chaitow and Sandy Fritz is a valuable and timely contribution to the field of manual therapy. I predict that almost every reader of this book will find new information and innovative methods for developing their hands-on skills and enhancing their clinical outcomes. This book is articulate, detailed, sequential, profoundly instructive and breathtakingly thorough.

Trigger point approaches consistently yield powerful therapeutic results. Stubborn cases of thoracic outlet are successfully resolved by neutralizing scalene and pectoralis minor trigger points. Trochanteric bursitis, all too often injected with cortisone (yielding little long-term success), is often cleared within three visits of treating quadratus lumborum and vastus lateralis trigger points. The sensation of having an ice pick in the mid-thoracic region upon deep inhalation is eradicated with trigger point work on the serratus posterior superior. 'Brain pain' from sub-occipital trigger points is effectively treated by normalizing tender points and hypertonicity in rectus capitis posterior minor and the adjacent sub-occipitals. The chronically stiff neck is significantly relieved by trapezius and levator scapula trigger point therapy. Deactivating trigger points as part of a whole body soft tissue approach is now a commonly accepted therapeutic modality.

Even today, Swedish Massage, or more appropriately Relaxation Therapy, is the primary reason why clients seek the services of massage therapists at our school clinic in Chicago. Clients intuitively know they need to relax, and that relaxation is profoundly therapeutic. But they want something more: 'could you spend a little more time on the back of my neck' or 'I strained my back pushing a piano last week' or 'I twisted a rib muscle while lifting my dog' or 'I'm just beginning a new job and find it painful to take a deep breath'. These are all indicators that the public wants, and expects, the massage session to be tailored to their personal needs: their familiar aches, pains and areas of dysfunction and stress. This book will significantly help to fill that gap.

A Massage Therapist's Guide to Understanding, Locating and Treating Myofascial Trigger Points features a thorough discussion of myofascial and other forms of pain and how stress can exacerbate pain symptoms. Causal factors and pain aetiology are presented and range from postural compensations to the chronic somatization described so vividly by Latey and others. Upper- and lower-crossed syndromes are discussed, providing regional, not just local, assessments of altered physiology, pain and dysfunction. Theories of trigger point development explain the evolution of this phenomenon and charts, maps and illustrations provide the visual learner with important clues to palpation accuracy.

Palpation for practitioners will assume a new dimension after reading this book. Texture, temperature, tonicity, trophic skin changes, attachments and musculotendinous junctions assume new clinical significance. Pressing, frictioning, stretching and direct pressure are but a few of the manual methods presented in order to detect deep, hidden, cryptic areas of longstanding pain.

As a massage therapy practitioner for the past three decades, what I find most important is how trigger point protocols can be incorporated into basic massage protocols and sequences. The implications of this are enormous. At health clubs, spas and resorts, the public can now expect a multi-dimensional approach to healing that combines the relaxation response with trigger point release techniques. This is a union long overdue!

The deactivation of pain-causing trigger points is both a science and an elegant art form. Congratulations to authors Chaitow and Fritz for an innovative contribution to this marriage of science and art.

Robert K. King, Founder & Past President,
Chicago School of Massage Therapy, 2006

Preface

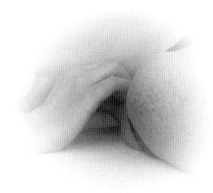

It has become ever more obvious that trigger points produce a great deal of the pain being treated by massage and manual therapists.

One of the main problems busy therapists face is keeping up to date with research evidence that explains the way trigger points develop, the way they create pain and dysfunction, and the best ways of deactivating them.

This book has been compiled precisely to meet that need; to help the therapist and the student to have a clear idea of what research and clinical experience has taught us in recent years.

To effectively manage trigger points it is necessary to know:

- why trigger points develop (see Chapters 1 and 2)
- where they develop (see Chapters 1 and 2)
- the nature and behavior of trigger points (see Chapter 3)
- the difference between active, latent, central, embryonic and attachment points – and why you need to know about these differences (see Chapters 1, 2 and 3)
- how some pain can be confusing – and why you need to be aware of 'imposter' symptoms (see Chapter 4)
- how nutrition, postural and breathing habits, stress and other factors can contribute to trigger point development (see Chapter 2)
- what symptoms trigger points can cause, and how to assess the patient's pain (see Chapter 5)

- how to locate trigger points by palpation (see Chapter 6)
- how to locate trigger points by using 'pain maps' (see Chapter 4)
- how to know if trigger points are significant (are they part of the patient's problem?) once they have been located (see Chapters 2, 4 and 7)
- when trigger points can be seen as functionally useful – for example if they are close to an unstable joint (see Chapter 7)
- how to deactivate trigger points using one of a variety of ways – including use of muscle energy, positional release, spray and stretch, and many more (see Chapter 7)
- how to integrate the methods described (and others) into a massage context (see Chapter 8)
- what other methods exist for treating trigger points outside of a massage therapist's scope of practice (see Chapter 9)
- what to advise the patient regarding home management methods (see Chapter 7).

Trigger points are almost always a part of the story in chronic pain settings, and major research has demonstrated the value of massage in treatment of chronic pain. Much of this research will be described throughout the book.

By understanding and managing myofascial trigger points effectively you can relieve a great deal of pain safely, and enhance the wellbeing of your patients.

Leon Chaitow, 2006

Acknowledgements

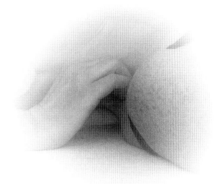

I wish to pay tribute to the work of a remarkable man, David Simons, whose half-century of dedicated research into myofascial pain continues unabated in his ninth decade. Special thanks also to my co-author Sandy Fritz for her unfailing contribution of time and effort, when there were already great demands on her both personally and professionally. However my primary thanks are to my wife Alkmini. Neither this book, nor any others to which I have contributed, would exist were it not for the supportive and loving safe haven that she has created in our home on the remarkable island of Corfu, Greece.

CHAPTER ONE

Myofascial and other pain

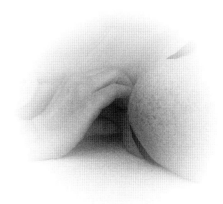

Pain is unpleasant, both physically and emotionally, and the more anxious a person is about a pain, the worse the pain will seem.

Pain is by far the commonest reason for anyone seeking advice and/or help from a healthcare provider – whether mainstream or complementary, and low back pain is the second most common reason for anyone consulting a physician in the USA (Merskey & Bogduk 1994).

We feel most pain in our muscles, fascia, ligaments, etc., the soft parts of the musculoskeletal system, which is the body's largest organizational system, and its greatest energy user (Deyo & Weinstein 2001).

It is this system, under the control of the nervous system, that supports, stabilizes and moves the joints and bones of the body, allowing us to walk, talk, dance, run, type and to generally express our human condition (Korr 1986).

This is why pain or dysfunction in the musculo-skeletal system has the ability to impact on our lives so greatly.

For more than any other reason, pain takes people to a physician or other healthcare provider, for help and advice. Pain can be mysterious, with no obvious cause, and this is the most worrying of all. Imagination can take hold, and an ache that is the result of nothing more than poor posture can escalate into something very serious in the person's mind.

This sort of 'catastrophizing' is even more likely when pain is felt in an area where there really is nothing 'wrong'. A pain in the face and head might be the direct result of a trigger point in the muscles of the neck area (such as upper trapezius or sternomastoid) – but because the pain is in the face, around the ear, or in the eyes, it is in those areas that the sufferer might imagine serious problems to exist.

Understanding that the pain is actually in the neck and shoulder muscles, removes the anxiety. After that, all that needs to be done is to deactivate the trigger points (see Chapter 7) and to see what can be done to prevent the same postural stresses from creating new ones!

Whether pain in soft tissues arises because of overload, overuse or injury, there is a strong chance that part of the pain process will involve the presence of hyperirritable areas of tissue known as myofascial trigger points (Wall & Melzack 1990).

- A myofascial trigger point is a hyperirritable spot, usually lying within a taut band of skeletal muscle, or in the muscle's fascia.
- This irritable spot (trigger point) will be painful on pressure, and often gives rise to referred or radiating pain and tenderness (Simons et al 1999)
- Chronic strain can affect any of the body's skeletal muscles, and so any muscle can develop myofascial trigger points.
- Myofascial pain syndromes are conditions of widespread pain that are both caused and maintained by one or more active trigger points.
- While the trigger point is the actual pain generator that causes the pain, other factors are the cause of the trigger point's activities.
- This makes it obvious that getting rid of myofascial pain requires that we either get rid of the trigger point(s) or the reasons for their existence.

Trigger points, what causes them, and the problems they can cause, will be described in detail in this and the next two chapters.

ACUTE AND CHRONIC PAIN

One definition of acute pain is that it is new, of recent onset (a matter of weeks) (Kolt & Andersen 2004). Another definition is that, even if not new, pain may be so severe as to be described as acute, even though it has been present for some time.

Acute pain usually involves a degree of tissue damage, and starts with what is called a phasic response. There may or may not be a verbal 'ouch', but there will almost always be a non-verbal response – for example contorting the face, or swiftly taking a hand away from a flame (Kolt & Andersen 2004).

The acute phase of a painful experience involves increased sympathetic nervous system activity, the degree of which is directly linked to how much fear or anxiety is associated with the pain (Craig 1994, Crombez 1998).

Pain in general – particularly acute pain – frequently has protective value, preventing the use of an area that has been injured, so allowing a period of rest for normal recovery to take place – after a strain, for example.

But even when pain does not last for very long, and although it may be useful in a protective way, it is not pleasant. However, such pain will have a meaning, it needs to be understood.

And pain that you understand is easier to cope with than pain that is mysterious, of unknown origin, and that feels threatening (Wall & Melzack 1990).

Chronic pain is generally defined as having been present for months rather than weeks. Chronic pain usually has a different character, compared to acute pain, aching and deep, rather than sharp or burning – although this is not always the case – for there are hundreds of words used to describe the quality of a pain (Wall & Melzack 1990).

The ache of chronic pain may be linked to the increased sympathetic tone that started as an acute episode (after lifting, for example), but which continues long after the healing of tissue damage has taken place.

This continuation of pain may increase levels of anxiety, fear and/or depression – especially if the reasons for the pain are not understood, or if treatment fails to ease the pain (Craig 1994).

It is important for therapists and practitioners to be able to explain to their clients/patients the probable cause(s) of any pain that is being experienced, and what can be done about it, using language that is simple yet accurate.

This is particularly true of pain deriving from myofascial trigger points, about which the public knows relatively little.

PAIN THAT STARTS SLOWLY

Pain does not always start as an acute experience, of course.

It sometimes develops slowly, starting as discomfort, only gradually becoming really painful over a period of months or years, as a result of such factors as poor posture, overuse, under-exercising (deconditioning), etc.

The process of slow-onset, microtrauma-induced dysfunction often includes the development of irritable, extremely sensitive areas in the soft tissues, known as myofascial trigger points (Simons et al 1999).

The pain symptoms associated with different types of trigger points, active, latent, embryonic, etc. are described in Box 1.1, while their special characteristics are outlined in Chapters 2 and 3.

PAIN IN CONTEXT

Pain and restriction should be seen in relation to the degree of acuteness or chronicity.

- Is it new? Has it been present for days, weeks, months or years? Has it changed recently? If so why?

Pain should also be seen in its association with the rest of the body.

- Is it worse/better when standing, sitting, lying … and if so why?
- What movements or other parts of the body seem to influence the pain?

It is also necessary to take account of the emotional and nutritional status, as well as the multiple environmental, occupational, social and other factors that affect the person.

- Are you settled in your work, relationships, home life, economically?
- Do you eat a balanced diet, drink enough water, get enough sleep, exercise? Do you have any habits that might be negatively influencing your health (smoking, alcohol)?
- Are you taking any prescription medication?

A patient who is enduring social, economic and emotional worries, who is not getting enough exercise or sleep, whose diet is problematic … and who happens to report muscular pain and backache, is likely to achieve only short-term benefit from manual

Box 1.1   Pain characteristics of different types of trigger points: active, latent, embryonic and satellite (Kuchera 1997, Simons et al 1999, Travell & Simons 1992)

NOTE: The full list of the characteristics of trigger points is to be found in Chapter 2; this list only looks at the different types of pain and sensation characteristics of the three main types of trigger point: active, latent and embryonic.

The pain characteristics of an active myofascial trigger point are:
- The area in which an active trigger point is located may already be sensitive before it is touched.
- When pressure is applied active trigger points are painful and either refer (i.e. symptoms are felt at a distance from the point of pressure) or radiate (i.e. symptoms spread from the point of pressure).
- Symptoms that are referred or radiated include pain, tingling, numbness, burning, itching or other sensations, and most importantly, these symptoms are recognizable (familiar) to the person.
- There are other signs of an active trigger point ('jump sign', palpable indications such as a taut band, fasciculation, etc.) and these will be described in Chapter 2.

Questions asked on application of pressure are:
1. 'Does this hurt?'
2. 'Does this hurt anywhere other than where I am pressing?'
3a. 'Do you recognize the pain?' or
3b 'Is this the pain you have been experiencing?'

If the answers to questions 1, 2 and 3 are all 'yes', this is an *active myofascial trigger point.*

The pain characteristics of a latent myofascial trigger point are:
- Commonly the individual is not aware of the existence of a latent point until it is pressed (that is, unlike an active point, a latent one seldom produces spontaneous pain).
- When pressure is applied to a latent point it is usually painful, and it may refer (i.e. symptoms are felt at a distance from the point of pressure), or radiate (i.e. symptoms spread from the point of pressure).
- If the symptoms, whether pain, tingling, numbness, burning, itching or other sensations, *are not familiar,* or perhaps are sensations that the person used to have in

the past, but has not experienced recently, then this is a *latent myofascial trigger point.*

The questions asked of the patient are of course the same, but if the answers to questions 1 and 2 are 'yes', and the answer to question 3 is 'no', the point is defined as latent, not active.

Progression from latent to active
Latent trigger points may become active trigger points at any time, perhaps becoming a 'common, everyday headache' or adding to, or expanding, the pattern of pain already being experienced for other reasons.

The change from latent to active may occur when the tissues are overused, strained by overload, chilled, stretched (particularly if this is rapid), shortened, traumatized (as in a motor vehicle accident or a fall or blow) or when other perpetuating factors (such as poor nutrition or shallow breathing) provide less than optimal conditions for tissue health.

Active trigger points may become latent trigger points with their referral patterns subsiding for brief or prolonged periods of time. They may then be reactivated with their referral patterns returning for no apparent reason.

Embryonic points
Any sensitive point in the soft tissues that hurts unusually on pressure, but which does not radiate or refer, is termed an *embryonic* trigger point.
This is a disturbed or dysfunctional region of soft tissue that, over time, with sufficient additional stress input (overuse, etc.), may become first a latent, and eventually, an active trigger point.

Embryonic points may evolve in the referral or radiation zone (the area influenced by an active or latent point – see above for descriptions of these). In that case the new, potential, trigger is known as a *satellite* point.

When a trigger point is situated near the center (belly) of a muscle, near the motor endpoint, it is known as a central point. When it is situated close to the insertion/attachment of a muscle, it is known as an *attachment* point. These are treated quite differently because of the characteristics of the tissues in which they lie. This will be fully explained in Chapter 7.

treatment if no account is taken of the many stresses being experienced.

What would often help most may not be possible: a new job, a new home, a new spouse (or removal of the present one), for example.

In such cases the therapist may at best be able to reduce the intensity of a patient's symptoms, but not be able deal with causes.

Or there may be a variety of simple changes that are possible – improved exercise and sleep patterns, better diet and stress management (relaxation and breathing exercises perhaps). If advice on such changes can be given, manual treatment of pain and dysfunction is likely to be more successful.

The lesson this offers is that dealing with the obvious (symptoms such as pain) may only be part of what is needed; the context, the background, often also needs attention.

And of course referral to specialist healthcare providers is the best choice where background causes are beyond the scope of practice of a therapist.

WHAT IS FACILITATION?

Trigger points can be described as 'locally facilitated' areas (Korr 1978, 1981).

Facilitation (or sensitization) involves pain-reporting (nociceptive) nerve cells (neurons) that are maintained in a hyperirritable state (Patterson 1976).

Nerve cells become sensitized when they have been repeatedly irritated.

Once nerve cells are sensitized they will be affected by even low levels of additional irritation.

This process is called 'facilitation' in osteopathic medicine (Korr 1986).

Facilitation/sensitization can take place in spinal soft tissues (where the process is known as 'segmental facilitation'), or it can occur in soft tissues anywhere else in the body, in the form of myofascial trigger points.

In some cases spinal (segmental) facilitation is the result of organ dysfunction or disease. For example, a facilitated area in the upper back (thoracic spinal levels 2 to 5) may be the result of heart problems, where 'feedback' to the spine along the nerve tracts that service the heart are responsible for the irritation of that area. This does not mean that treating the spinal segment could influence heart disease, but that the facilitated area is likely to remain a problem for as long as the heart is a problem (Kuchera 1997). See Figure 1.1.

The causes of increased sensitivity/facilitation can also include overuse of an area through persistent habitual patterns of use, posture, etc.

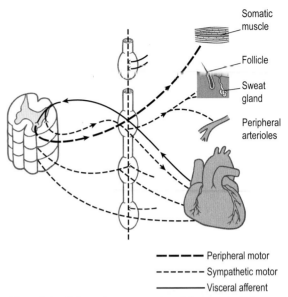

Figure 1.1   Schematic representation of the neurological influences involved in the process of facilitation resulting from visceral dysfunction (cardiac disease in this example). Hyperirritable neural feedback to the CNS will result, which influences muscle, skin (both palpable) and venous structures in associated areas, as well as the neural supply to the organ itself. (From Chaitow 2001.)

Areas of facilitation, whether local trigger points or spinal segments, have a different 'feel' (congested, indurated, fibrous/'stringy', tense, etc.) and will also usually be sensitive and be less flexible/elastic.

As will become clear in Chapter 6, these feelings of being 'different' from surrounding, more normal tissues are very useful when trying to identify trigger points.

EDEMA AND TRIGGER POINT SENSITIZATION

A part of the process that encourages facilitation of local nerve structures, leading to increasing sensitivity and pain, involves the release of irritating chemicals, as described below.

A sequence is thought to take place as follows (Mense & Simons 2001):

- 'Something happens' to muscle tissue – this could be a sudden strain, or a blow, a chill, a rapid stretch, or a series of repetitive micro-injuries brought about by overuse, for example.
- The 'something' that happens causes the release of highly irritating chemicals.

- These include *vaso-neuro-reactive* substances (such as bradykinin, prostaglandin, interleukin-1 and substance P – see Box 2.4, Chapter 2 for more about these chemicals and how they help create trigger points).
- These chemicals increase the sensitivity of local nerve cells that report pain to the central nervous system and brain (called nociceptors).
- These chemicals also cause the local blood vessels to swell, and encourage increased permeability (the ease with which substances can pass through their walls), creating localized swelling, congestion, edema.
- The swollen tissues press on tiny blood vessels and reduce the free flow of blood, causing ischemia (literally 'lack of blood').
- Because of ischemia there will be reduced oxygen levels in the tissues.
- Tissues depend on oxygen to function, and to be able to produce energy.
- Ischemia increases the release of substance P, and this adds to the irritation of nerve structures.
- After a while the pain-receptor nerve cells (nociceptors) will become sensitized, and will have a reduced tolerance/threshold, making them more easily irritated than before.
- Imagine the loudspeaker of a hi-fi system on which the volume has been turned up, so that what was previously heard as low level sound is now very loud.
- This is how a sensitized, facilitated, pain receptor behaves, amplifying the messages being received, and sometimes misinterpreting non-pain messages as pain.
- Discomfort becomes soreness, soreness becomes pain, and pain becomes agony.
- Increased sympathetic activity in the person ('stress', fear, alarm, etc.) causes release of a variety of other substances, such as norepinephrine (noradrenaline).
- The now oversensitive pain receptors find this irritating, causing even more pain messages to be sent to the central nervous system (CNS), and brain.
- The pain itself will often become a source of new anxiety and stress, making the whole process worse.

Details of the series of events that is thought to take place in tissues when a trigger point forms will be described in later chapters. See Box 2.4 in Chapter 2, which describes the results of remarkable recent research that has analyzed the tissues of trigger points, and Figure 1.2.

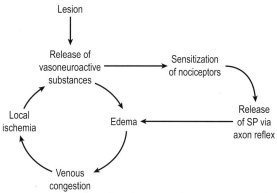

Figure 1.2 Hypothetical mechanism explaining tenderness of myofascial trigger points. (Reproduced with permission, from Mense S & Simons D *Muscle Pain*, Lippincott Williams & Wilkins, 2001.)

OTHER INFLUENCES

Apart from overuse and trauma, it is known that high levels of emotional, and psychological distress, as well as background chemical changes (e.g. iron deficiency or hormonal imbalance), will also encourage sensitization (Simons et al 1999).

Many of these processes are discussed further in Chapters 2 and 3 (see also Box 1.2).

Ideally the background causes of trigger points and facilitation should be removed or reduced, but because this may take time, treatment to ease the pain and other symptoms is commonly called for, by deactivation of active trigger points (Fig. 1.3).

The choice of methods used to deactivate an active trigger point depends on the training and licensing status of the practitioner/therapist, and will be described in detail in Chapters 7, 8 and 9.

STRESS REACTION

When an area is facilitated, whether 'segmentally' alongside the spine, or in muscle or fascia (trigger point), there will be increased neural activity (and therefore more pain) when either the area itself – or the body as a whole – is stressed, in any way.

In this way a trigger point behaves like 'neurological lenses'. Korr (1986) used this metaphor because he compared the way a trigger point can 'focus' (or amplify) any general stress, through itself, in much the same way that a magnifying glass focuses sunlight to a tiny point (Fig. 1.4).

When there is physical, environmental or psychological stress, such as we all experience in our daily lives (deadlines, traffic jams, other people's

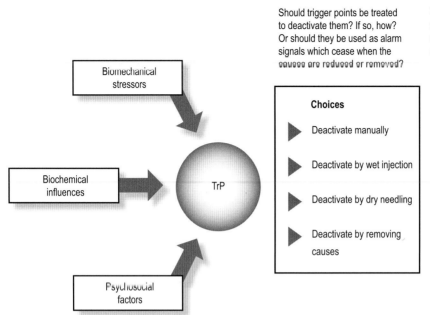

Should trigger points be treated to deactivate them? If so, how? Or should they be used as alarm signals which cease when the causes are reduced or removed?

Figure 1.3   Schematic representation of trigger point deactivation choices. (From Chaitow 2003.)

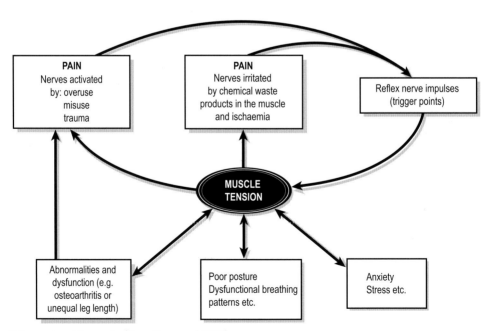

Figure 1.4   Pain–tension vicious cycle. (From Peters et al 2002.)

behavior, financial or domestic worries, exams, etc.) there will be increased neural activity (sympathetic responses) in the local areas (such as trigger points) that have become sensitized.

Trigger points can therefore be understood to be in a virtually permanent state of 'physiological alarm'.

This means that any methods that produce relaxation and calm, that reduce sympathetic arousal, are likely to result in less pain being sensed from the activity of trigger points.

This is supported by research that shows that relaxation massage – or anything else that has a calming effect – does precisely this, reducing pain deriving from trigger points (de las Peñas 2005). This will become clearer in Chapter 7, where treatment options are outlined.

A definition of stress, and the way it affects the body, is explained in Box 1.2.

Box 1.2   Understanding stress and adaptation

Stress can be defined as anything that makes a demand on the body to adapt. Stress can also be seen as any physical or mental challenge that provokes a response in the body that enables a person to meet the challenge, or to flee from it.

The responses of the body will be different, depending on whether the adaptation demand (stress) is a single event, or a series of events that are either continuous or repetitive.

A single alarm reaction to a demand ('fight or flight') will produce an acute response, with increased heart rate, blood pressure, muscle tone, etc., as the body prepares for instant action – this is also known as *sympathetic arousal*.

If the same, or other, demands are ongoing or repetitive, the 'alarm' stage gives way to the stage of resistance, or adaptation. When this happens, although there seems to be better coping with the original stress, this is – according to Selye's research – at the expense of the ability to handle other stresses (Selye 1974).

As a person accommodates and adapts to any stressor, other stressors require lower thresholds to trigger alarm reactions.

Selye also showed that when there are a number of stressors at the same time this triggers an alarm reaction even though the individual stress factors on their own would not have had this effect. Take for example a person who is trying to multi-task, is overloaded both physically and emotionally, is already in pain, has not had enough sleep, and who is low in blood sugar because meals are being skipped; each 'stress factor' on its own could be coped with, but when they all exist together, a state of sympathetic arousal, anxiety and increased sensitivity would exist.

To use a different, chemical, example: if someone was exposed to one-third of a dose of histamine, together with one-third of a dose of exposure to extreme cold, plus one-third of a dose of formaldehyde, an alarm reaction would occur, equal to a full dose of any one of these stressors.

So it seems that as adaptation to life's stresses and stressors continues, thresholds drop so that even a slight stress factor is capable of producing a reaction – pain for example – from facilitated structures, whether these are paraspinal or myofascial.

We all adapt to repetitive activity. The letters SAID (specific adaptation to imposed demand) describe the changes that occur in the body in response to particular activities (Norris 2000).

This process of adaptation applies to activities such as athletic or weight training, as well as to any regularly performed task or activity, such as playing an instrument, typing on a keyboard, using a work- or hobby-related tool, digging a garden, or any other prolonged or repetitive activity.

But our potential for adaptation is limited – by age, physical condition, previous trauma, nutritional status and many other factors.

After a period of adaptation that may last for many years (following the initial alarm reaction), when the limits of adaptation are reached, tissues break down.

This is known as the stage of collapse, or exhaustion, and is when major symptoms may appear (joint damage for example).

Like a piece of elastic that has reached its limits, particular tissues may just not be able to cope with whatever stresses they are being asked to handle. (Fig. 1.5.)

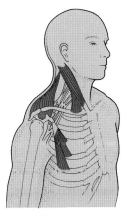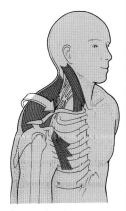

Figure 1.5   A progressive pattern of postural and biomechanical dysfunction develops, resulting in, and aggravated by, inappropriate breathing function. (From Chaitow 2001.)

Box 1.2   Understanding stress and adaptation – *cont'd*

A formula for recovery

When we are examining a person, or a part (shoulder, knee, etc.) it is worth considering the following questions:

- How well is the person or the part adapting to the demands being imposed?
- How much adaptive potential remains?
- How close to exhaustion is this shoulder?
- How near to adaptive exhaustion is this person?

Helping to stop or slow down degeneration, delaying adaptive exhaustion, involves one of two options:

- improve the ability of the person, or tissues, to handle the stress load, or
- reduce or eliminate the load.

MORE ON THE PAIN PROCESS

Unfortunately pain is not always useful as a warning, and sometimes it does not stop on its own.

Chronic pain may sometimes be part of a process left over from a past event, such as surgery (scar tissues often have trigger points alongside – see Chapter 4), major trauma (whiplash, fracture, etc.), or serious pathology such as degenerative arthritis or cancer.

In such situations pain may be of little value as an alarm, and indeed in many chronic pain situations the continuous, or intermittent yet persistent, nature of the pain – whether it involves sensations that are aching, burning, searing, stabbing, etc. – creates additional problems.

The pain may lead to emotional or physical symptoms, interfering with movement and sleep, and generally preventing performance of the normal activities of life.

Myofascial trigger points are almost always a part of such chronic, widespread pain and dysfunction, and while deactivating them may not change the underlying serious condition, it can reduce pain levels, making life more tolerable (Wall & Melzack 1990).

DECOMPENSATION

Grieve (1986) has clearly described a common sequence that relates to patients presenting with pain or restricted movement.

- The person may have suffered a major injury that has overwhelmed the tolerances of relatively healthy tissues (muscles, ligaments, joints).
- Or the individual will show signs of gradual decompensation, because of slow exhaustion of the tissue's adaptive potential, for example through overuse, with or without trauma.
- As this process of decompensation continues there will, over time, be other changes that can lead to exhaustion of the body's adaptive potential, with more pain and restriction as a result.

- Think of the example of someone with a simple problem such as a heel-spur, causing pain when standing on the affected leg.
- There will be a compensating way of standing and walking, with weight thrown onto the other side.
- Over time – and this can mean many years – excessive wear and tear on the other leg, possibly the hip, knee, low back, upper back or even neck, will start to produce symptoms of stiffness and pain.
- And there will be new compensations for these changes as well … and in the end the problem in the heel may be the background cause of widespread pain throughout the body.

A similar pattern of compensation and decompensation could just as easily be the result of an unbalanced temporomandibular joint, or any other part of the body that calls for compensating use patterns.

Whether a patient's problem involves chronic headache, jaw and/or facial pain, neck, shoulder and/or arm discomfort or pain, or back and/or pelvic pain, aching limbs, pain in the chest or abdomen, there is a strong likelihood that at least some, and sometimes almost all, of the pain will be deriving from the presence of active myofascial trigger points, possibly resulting from decompensation (Wall & Melzack 1990) (Fig. 1.6).

NOT JUST PAIN – FUNCTION AS WELL

Recent research has shown that trigger points that are not sufficiently sensitized to produce pain (such as latent trigger points – see Box 1.1 for an explanation) nevertheless interfere with normal muscle function (Lucas et al 2004).

It was shown that when there were latent trigger points (i.e. not producing any pain until pressed, and even then the pain was not a symptom the person recognized) in upper trapezius muscles (one of the commonest places for triggers, along with quadratus lumborum), there was a change in the way the other arm muscles behaved when the arm was raised.

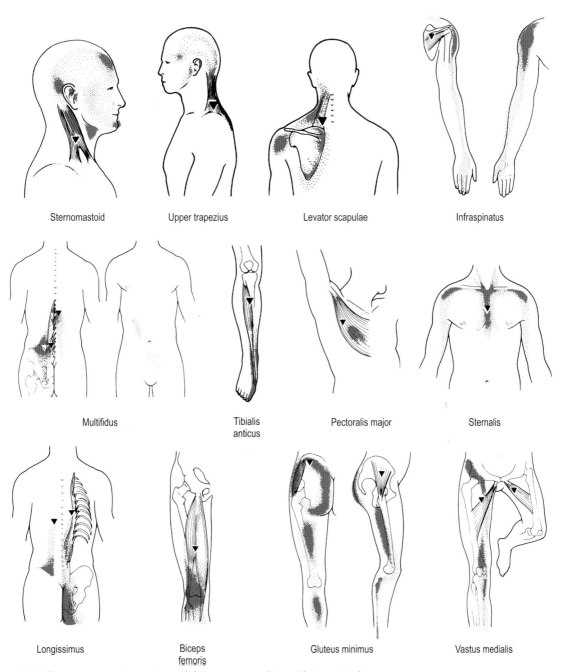

Figure 1.6   Some common trigger points and their target areas. (From Chaitow 2003.)

If the same sort of interference with the normal firing sequence of muscles occurred in, for example, the lower back muscles, this would significantly interfere with normal spinal stability.

CAN TRIGGER POINTS EVER BE USEFUL?

Trigger points modify the tone of the muscles in which they are located, and when trigger points refer or radiate pain, or other symptoms, into target areas (referral zones – see Box 1.1), the tone (tension, stiffness) of the muscle in these zones also changes (it usually increases).

If a person has genetically acquired laxity (looseness) of their ligaments they will be hyper-mobile and joints (such as the sacroiliac) will be relatively less stable than they should be, and overlying muscles will be obliged to increase activity to help maintain stability (Keer & Grahame 2003).

It is well known that hypermobile individuals are more prone to musculoskeletal problems such as back and sacroiliac pain and dysfunction (Bridges et al 1992).

Hypermobile people are also very prone to developing fibromyalgia, characterized by chronic body-wide pain symptoms (Gedalia et al 1993, Goldman 1991), and are also known to have an excessive number of active trigger points, compared with people who are not hypermobile (Simons et al 1999).

It seems reasonable to believe that, in a person who is hypermobile, trigger points, and the increased muscle tone they produce, may be functional, actually assisting in maintaining stability.

It is useful to consider that there may be times when deactivation of trigger points (as detailed in Chapters 7, 8 and 9) may not be in the best interests of the patient.

See Box 1.3 for an example of a 'useful' trigger point.

An alternative way of handling trigger points in someone who is hypermobile may be to use toning and conditioning exercises to improve the ability to stabilize whatever may be unstable, so reducing the need for trigger point activity.

TRIGGER POINTS AS MONITORS OF PROGRESS

At times it is possible to remove the reason for trigger point activity.

An example of this comes from a New Zealand physical therapist, specializing in breathing retraining. Dinah Bradley (2002) reports that before teaching breathing exercises to people with an upper chest pattern, she looks for trigger points in their intercostal muscles (Fig. 1.8). Having located several, she tests how much pressure is needed to produce pain in these points (using a pressure gauge/algometer – see Chapter 5 for more about this useful little instrument).

She then teaches the patient a home-breathing rehabilitation regime, and when she next sees the patient, some weeks later, she retests the amount of pressure needed to 'fire' the trigger points.

If the trigger points now require much more pressure to produce pain than they did when she first evaluated them, she is reassured that the person is doing their home-work, and that these intercostal muscles are less stressed, and that the trigger points in them will therefore be calmer (see Chapter 5 for discussion of pressure and pain levels).

This 'functional' approach to using trigger points recognizes the 'alarm' function they represent. By taking away the reason for their overactivity, by virtually 'putting out the fire', the alarms have stopped ringing.

Unfortunately this scenario is not true for all (or even most) trigger points because causes are not always easy to identify, and therefore change.

But when trigger points are possibly useful, or are capable of being deactivated by improved function (through postural reeducation, better use of the body, better breathing patterns, etc.), the therapeutic choices should reflect this.

OTHER SYMPTOMS THAN PAIN

Trigger points can be responsible for a wide variety of symptoms other than pain.

The major researchers into myofascial trigger point activity, Travell and Simons (Simons et al 1999, Travell & Simons 1992), have shown that trigger points interfere with normal secretions in the areas they influence. In this way skin changes, as well as, for example, digestive function can be altered by active or latent trigger point activity, and improved by their removal.

The influences of trigger points other than pain are listed in Box 1.4. See also Figures 1.9, 1.10, 1.11 and 1.12 in Box 1.4.

WHAT WE STILL NEED TO EXPLORE

The coming chapters will contain:

- Chapter 2: The biomechanical, psychological and biochemical processes – large and small – that allow trigger points to develop (such as poor posture, unbalanced breathing patterns, anxiety, overuse and misuse of muscles and joints, ischemia – poor blood and oxygen supply to the tissues, unbalanced nutrition and hormonal status, etc.).
- Chapter 3: More details about different types of points – particularly central and attachment points, and why it is important to know the difference, so that the central ones are chosen for first attention.
- Chapter 4: Maps, which parts of the body are affected by particular trigger points.
- Chapter 5: Assessing pain levels.
- Chapter 6: The many (and best) ways of palpating for, and locating trigger points.
- Chapter 7: How to choose where to start when there are many painful and active triggers (and which to leave alone because they might be useful), and the various ways in which they can be manually deactivated, including cryotherapy (spray and stretch), or be made to vanish without treatment

because the causes have been removed. Plus advice on preventing trigger points from recurring.

- Chapter 8: Managing trigger points in the context of a massage session.
- Chapter 9: Other methods of trigger point deactivation – such as use of magnets, lasers, ultrasound, thyroid hormone replacement, dry needling, analgesic injections and acupuncture. Some of these methods are used by licensed massage therapists (LMTs), but others require appropriate referral and licensure.

Box 1.3   Potentially useful trigger points

Symptoms are the signposts of adaptation.

Sometimes symptoms represent an adaptation failure (tissues unable to handle the stress and strain that is being imposed on them).

And sometimes symptoms represent adaptation in action.

Take, for example, the healing process following injury that involves inflammation.

Inflammation is a vital process of adaptation to tissue damage, without which the tissues could not heal.

And as we have seen, pain, hypertonicity and/or spasm can at times be protective.

Trigger points produce increased tone in the muscles housing them, as well as in tissues to which they refer, possibly offering an energy-efficient way of protecting a vulnerable joint (because trigger points are controlled by chemical processes, not nerves – as will be described in Chapter 2.)

For example:

- a gluteus maximus or latissimus dorsi trigger point would create increased tone in that muscle group, placing additional load on the thoracodorsal fascia, helping to protect an unstable sacroiliac joint (see Fig. 1.7B), or
- a trigger point in the hamstrings would increase tension on the sacrotuberous ligament, helping to protect an unstable sacroiliac joint (see biceps femoris trigger point in Fig. 1.6).

Not all trigger points are useful; many are residual evidence of past stresses, while newly developed triggers are often the result of the effects of currently active trigger points. See notes on satellite trigger points in Box 1.1 and the next chapters (Simons et al 1999).

It makes sense to attempt to remove the intensity of pain symptoms coming from a trigger point, but it makes more sense to focus on why the symptom exists, and to aim to remove or modify causes.

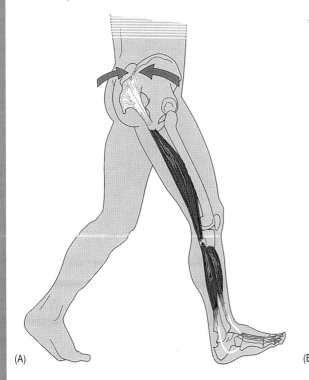

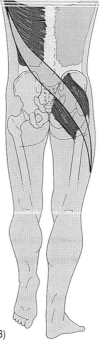

(A)   (B)

Figure 1.7   A: At heel strike, posterior rotation of the right innominate increases the tension of the right sacrotuberous ligament. Contraction of the biceps femoris further increases tension in this ligament, preparing the sacroiliac joint for impact. (Redrawn from Vleeming et al 1997.) B: During the right single-leg stance phase, contraction of the gluteus maximus and the contralateral latissimus dorsi increases tension through the thoracodorsal fascia and facilitates continued stability of the sacroiliac joint during the weight-bearing phase. (From Lee 1999.)

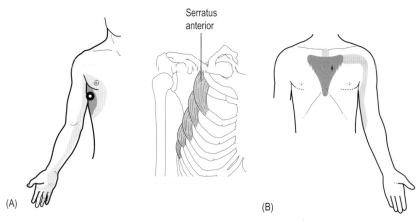

(A)   (B)

Figure 1.8   A: Serratus anterior trigger points include one which produces a 'short breath' condition as well as an often familiar interscapular pain. (From Chaitow & DeLany 2000). B: The pattern of pain referral from a trigger point (or points) in the sternalis muscle. (From Baldry 1993.)

Box 1.4   Trigger point symptoms other than pain (Kuchera 1997, Kuchera & McPartland 1997, Simons et al 1999, Slocumb 1984, Travell & Simons 1992, Weiss 2001)

- Appendicitis-like pain, usually during premenstrual phase of cycle (trigger point may be located at lower right margin of rectus abdominis muscle)
- Cardiac arrhythmias (trigger points in pectoralis major in particular)
- Colic – simulating abdominal or gallbladder symptoms (trigger point is close to costal margin, slightly left of center)
- Conjunctival reddening (trigger points in cervical or facial muscles)

- Dermatographia (trigger points referring to area where dermatographia is noted)
- Diarrhea, dysmenorrhea (trigger points in lower abdominal quadrants, left or right, often in lower rectus abdominis)
- Diminished gastric motility (trigger points in abdominal musculature)
- Excessive maxillary sinus secretion (trigger points in facial muscles)

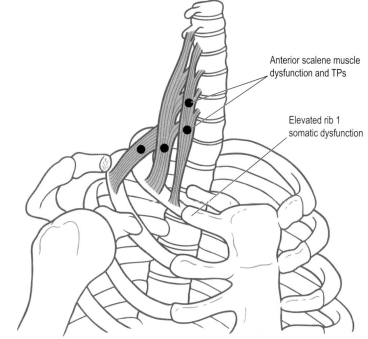

(A)

Figure 1.9   A: Location and B: effects of scalene trigger points. (Reproduced with permission, from Ward R (ed) *Foundations of Osteopathic Medicine*, Lippincott Williams & Wilkins, 1997.)

Box 1.4   Trigger point symptoms other than pain (Kuchera 1997, Kuchera & McPartland 1997, Simons et al 1999, Slocumb 1984, Travell & Simons 1992, Weiss 2001) – *cont'd*

- Gooseflesh (trigger points referring to area where gooseflesh is noted)
- Indigestion, nausea, 'heartburn' (trigger points in upper rectus abdominis – usually left side)
- Interstitial cystitis (trigger points located in lower abdomen, intrapelvic and inner thighs)
- Localized sweating (trigger points referring to area where sweating is noted)
- Proprioceptive disturbance, dizziness (trigger point is in cervical or facial muscles)

- Ptosis, excessive lacrimation (trigger points in facial muscles)
- Upper limb lymphatic stasis (trigger points in posterior axillary fold, and/or in lower aspect of anterior scalene)
- Urinary symptoms including spasm (trigger point immediately above symphysis pubis)
- Vasoconstriction and headache (trigger points lie in cervical or facial musculature)

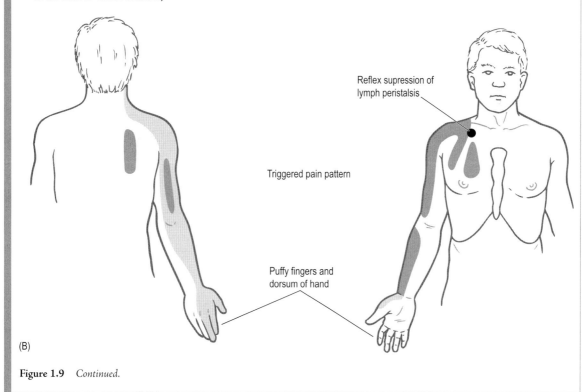

(B)

Figure 1.9   *Continued.*

Box 1.4   Trigger point symptoms other than pain (Kuchera 1997, Kuchera & McPartland 1997, Simons et al 1999, Slocumb 1984, Travell & Simons 1992, Weiss 2001) – *cont'd*

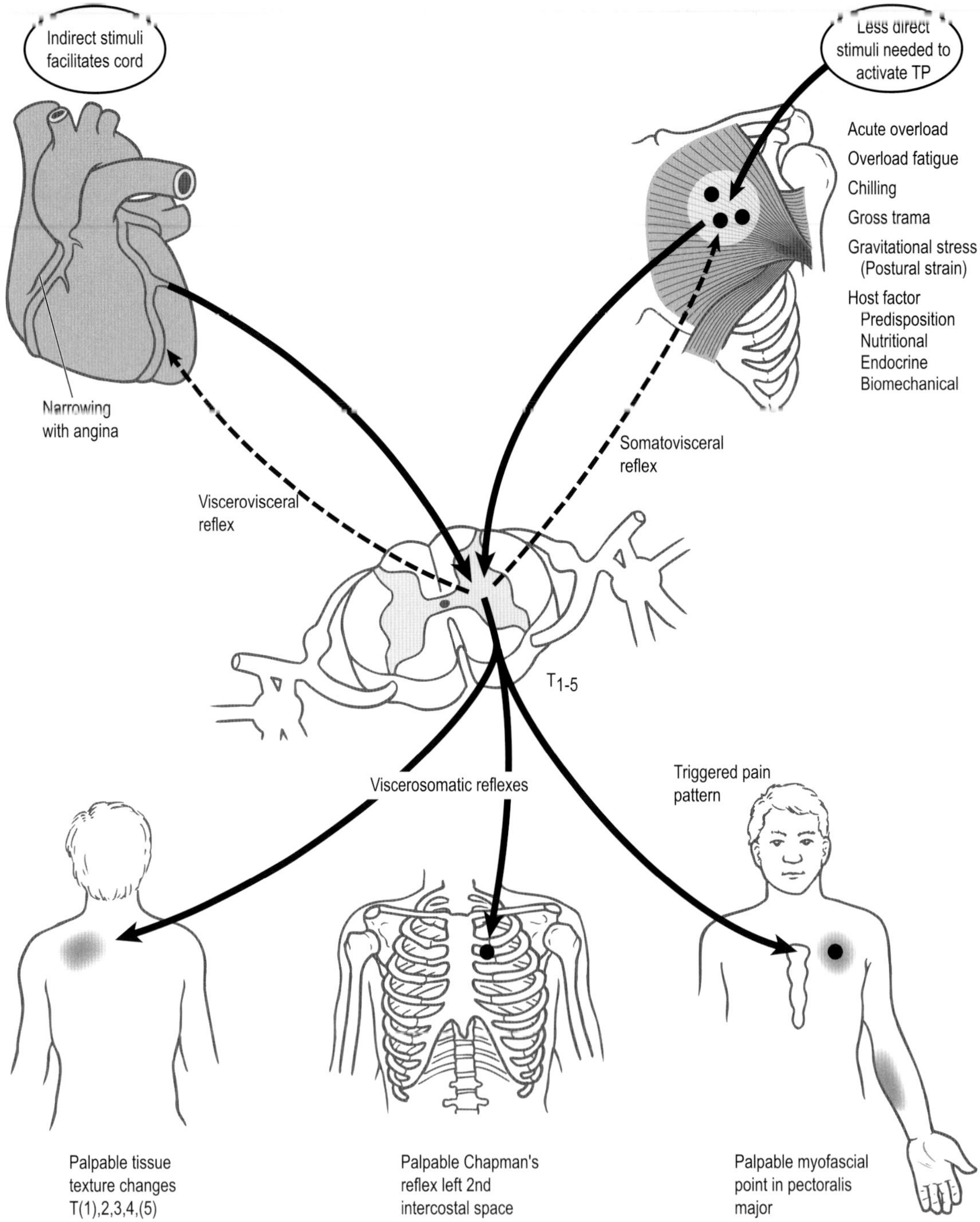

Indirect stimuli facilitates cord

Less direct stimuli needed to activate TP

Acute overload
Overload fatigue
Chilling
Gross trama
Gravitational stress (Postural strain)
Host factor
  Predisposition
  Nutritional
  Endocrine
  Biomechanical

Narrowing with angina

Somatovisceral reflex

Viscerovisceral reflex

T₁-₅

Viscerosomatic reflexes

Triggered pain pattern

Palpable tissue texture changes T(1),2,3,4,(5)

Palpable Chapman's reflex left 2nd intercostal space

Palpable myofascial point in pectoralis major

Figure 1.10   Spinal cord as organizer of disease processes. (Reproduced with permission, from Ward R (ed) *Foundations of Osteopathic Medicine*, Lippincott Williams & Wilkins, 1997.)

Box 1.4   Trigger point symptoms other than pain (Kuchera 1997, Kuchera & McPartland 1997, Simons et al 1999, Slocumb 1984, Travell & Simons 1992, Weiss 2001) – *cont'd*

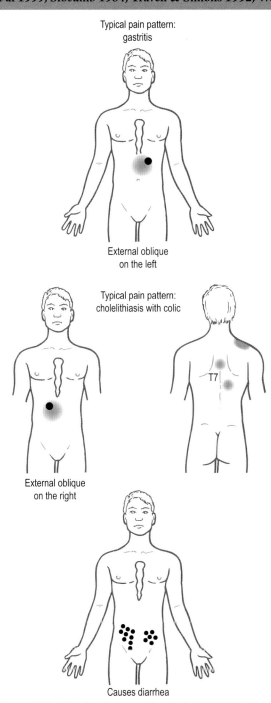

Typical pain pattern: gastritis

External oblique on the left

Typical pain pattern: cholelithiasis with colic

External oblique on the right

T7

Causes diarrhea

Figure 1.11   Myofascial trigger points and viscerosomatic reflexes. (Reproduced with permission, from Ward R (ed) *Foundations of Osteopathic Medicine*, Lippincott Williams & Wilkins, 1997.)

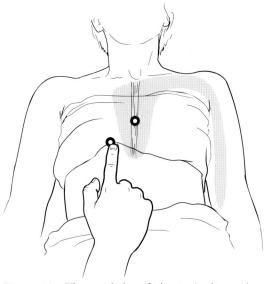

Figure 1.12   The sternalis has a frightening 'cardiac-type' pain pattern independent of movement while the cardiac arrhythmia trigger point (see fingertip) contributes to disturbances in normal heart rhythm without pain referral. (From Chaitow & DeLany 2000.)

CLINICAL NOTE

Key points from Chapter 1

1. There are different types of trigger points, but the most clinically important is an active point that produces symptoms that the patient recognizes.

2. Trigger points can produce many other symptoms than pain.

3. Trigger points are commonly part of most chronic pain problems, and at times may be the main source of the pain.

4. Trigger points are areas of facilitation, commonly emerging from a background of adaptation, or failure of adaptation.

5. Deactivating such triggers may not correct underlying conditions but can make life more tolerable by reducing the pain burden.

6. At times, trigger points may be performing a useful stabilizing function (always consider this if the person – or joint – is hypermobile).

7. Facilitated areas, such as trigger points, are easily aggravated by any form of stress (biochemical, biomechanical, psychosocial, climatic, etc.) affecting the body as a whole, as well as by local stress.

8. Removing the causes of trigger point activity is the best 'treatment', but if this is not possible deactivation can usually be achieved using manual and complementary methods.

References

Baldry P 1993 Acupuncture, trigger points and musculoskeletal pain. Churchill Livingstone, Edinburgh

Bradley D 2002 In: Chaitow L, Bradley D, Gilbert C Multidisciplinary approaches to breathing pattern disorders. Churchill Livingstone, Edinburgh, p 178

Bridges A, Smith E, Reid J 1992 Joint hypermobility in adults referred to rheumatology clinics. Annals of the Rheumatic Diseases 51:793–796

Chaitow L 2001 Muscle energy techniques, 2nd edn. Churchill Livingstone, Edinburgh

Chaitow L 2003 Modern neuromuscular techniques, 2nd edn. Churchill Livingstone, Edinburgh

Chaitow L, DeLany J 2000 Clinical applications of neuromuscular technique. Churchill Livingstone, Edinburgh

Chaitow L, Bradley D, Gilbert C 2002 Multidisciplinary approaches to breathing pattern disorders. Churchill Livingstone, Edinburgh

Craig K 1994 Emotional aspects of pain. In: Wall P, Melzack R (eds) Textbook of pain. Churchill Livingstone, Edinburgh, p 261–274

Crombez G 1998 When somatic information threatens, catastrophic thinking enhances attention interference. Pain 75:187–198

de las Peñas C-F 2005 Manual therapies in myofascial trigger point treatment: a systematic review. Journal of Bodywork and Movement Therapies 9(1):27–34

Deyo R, Weinstein J 2001 Low back pain. New England Journal of Medicine 344(5):363–369

Gedalia A, Press J, Klein M, Buskila D 1993 Joint hypermobility and fibromyalgia in schoolchildren. Annals of the Rheumatic Diseases 52:494–496

Goldman J 1991 Hypermobility and deconditioning: links to fibromyalgia. Southern Medical Journal 84:1192–1196

Grieve G 1986 Modern manual therapy. Churchill Livingstone, London

Keer R, Grahame R 2003 Hypermobility syndrome. Butterworth Heinemann, London, p 155–156

Kolt G Andersen M 2004 Psychology in the physical and manual therapies. Churchill Livingstone Edinburgh

Korr I (ed) 1978 Sustained sympatheticotonia as a factor in disease. In: The neurobiological mechanisms in manipulative therapy. Plenum Press, New York

Korr I M 1981 Spinal cord as organizer of disease processes. Journal of the American Osteopathic Association 80:451

Korr I M 1986 Somatic dysfunction, osteopathic manipulative treatment and the nervous system. Journal of the American Osteopathic Association 86(2):109–114

Kuchera M 1997 Travell & Simons Myofascial trigger points. In: Ward R (ed) Foundations for osteopathic medicine. Williams & Wilkins, Baltimore, p 919–933

Kuchera M, McPartland J 1997 Myofascial trigger points. In: Ward R (ed) Foundations for osteopathic medicine. Williams & Wilkins, Baltimore, p 915–918

Lee D G 1999 The pelvic girdle, 2nd edn. Churchill Livingstone, Edinburgh

Lucas K, Polus B I, Rich P A 2004 Latent myofascial trigger points: their effects on muscle activation and movement efficiency. Journal of Bodywork and Movement Therapies 8(3):160–166

Mense S, Simons D 2001 Muscle pain. Lippincott Williams & Wilkins, Philadelphia

Merskey H, Bogduk N 1994 Classification of chronic pain. Definitions of chronic pain syndromes and definition of chronic pain, 2nd edn. International Association for the Study of Pain, Seattle, WA

Norris C 2000 Back stability. Human Kinetics, Champaign, IL

Patterson M 1976 Model mechanism for spinal segmental facilitation. Academy of Applied Osteopathy Yearbook, Carmel, CA

Peters D, Chaitow L, Harris G, Morrison S 2002 Integrating complementary therapies into primary care. Churchill Livingstone, Edinburgh

Selye H 1974 Stress without distress. Lippincott, Philadelphia

Simons D, Travell J, Simons L 1999 Myofascial pain and dysfunction, 2nd edn. Upper body. Williams & Wilkins, Baltimore

Slocumb J 1984 Neurological factors in chronic pelvic pain trigger points and abdominal pelvic pain. American Journal of Obstetrics and Gynecology 49:536

Travell J, Simons D 1992 Myofascial pain and dysfunction. Lower body. Williams & Wilkins, Baltimore

Vleeming A, Mooney V, Dorman T et al 1997 Movement stability and low back pain: the essential role of the pelvis. Churchill Livingstone, Edinburgh

Wall P, Melzack R 1990 Textbook of pain, 2nd edn. Churchill Livingstone, Edinburgh

Ward R (ed) 1997 Foundations of osteopathic medicine. Williams & Wilkins, Baltimore

Weiss J 2001 Pelvic floor myofascial trigger points: manual therapy for interstitial cystitis and the urgency-frequency syndrome. Journal of Urology 166:2226–2231

CHAPTER TWO

How trigger points start – the big and the small picture

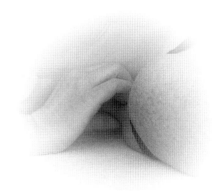

In Chapter 1 we saw that myofascial trigger points emerge from a background of dysfunction and adaptation.

In this chapter we will examine both the larger, and the smaller (cellular), processes that allow this to happen.

THE BIG PICTURE

To get a sense of the big picture an outline is given below of some of the major features that set the scene for trigger points to become active – including those that are mainly biomechanical, biochemical and/or psychological (and others such as climatic influences).

Causes of soft tissue distress and trigger point development

It's important to remember that problems of pain and dysfunction commonly (almost always in fact outside of direct physical trauma) have a combination of causes.

The list of interacting influences below offers a sample of the most obvious 'causes'. The fact is that few of these factors, on their own, could produce problems. But when you combine several of these features, the ability of the body, or the part (knee, shoulder, etc.) to cope, or to adapt, may start to break down.

One of your tasks as a manual therapist is to identify the contributing factors, and to help the person to either eliminate them, or to handle them better – as well as trying to ease the symptoms that have resulted.

Dealing with associated trigger points will often be a major part of that process.

The main influences on dysfunction can be described as being either congenital (inborn), or the result of overuse, misuse, abuse, disuse or of reflexive activity – or any combination of these.

Congenital – for example short leg, fascial distortion, hypermobility, etc. (Fig. 2.1A). Birth trauma, such as cranial injury from forceps or vacuum delivery, or even too short or too long a time in the birth canal, can distort the skull, including the internal cranial fascia, which, because of body-wide fascial continuity, can cause compensating distortions elsewhere in the body (Carriero 2003) (Fig. 2.1B).

Overuse/misuse – including poor postural, occupational and/or recreational habits possibly involving 'crossed syndrome patterns' (see below); and/or functional stress (e.g. upper chest breathing pattern). Postures and patterns that we adopt and use for many hours daily are prime suspects. We need to know how a person spends their day; how they sit (including details of what type of car they drive), walk, stand, perform work- and leisure-related tasks and movements – and for how long (Janda 1986, 1996) (Figs 2.1C and 2.1D).

Abuse – for example injury such as whiplash, surgery, repetitive use (microtrauma). It is important also to know what treatment if any the person had or is having (Fig. 2.1E).

Disuse – for example immobilization, inactivity, sedentary occupation, protective (as in arthritic joint or disc problems). Underactivity can be just as damaging as overactivity (Simons et al 1999).

Reflexive – for example facilitated segments, involving viscerosomatic influences (as described in Chapter 1, see Fig. 1.1) and trigger points that generate new

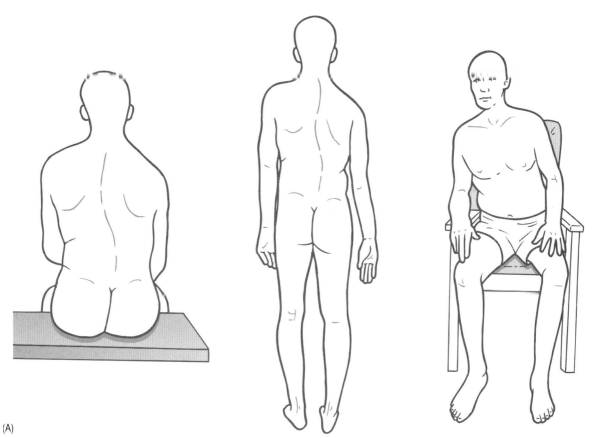

(A)

Figure 2.1A   Examples of common congenital structural imbalances which result in sustained functional/postural stress – small hemipelvis, short leg and short upper extremity. (From Chaitow 2001.)

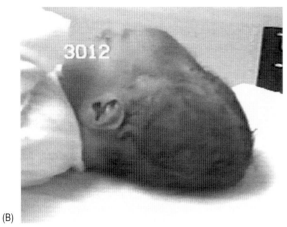

(B)

Figure 2.1B   A 6-hour-old newborn with extensive molding following prolonged labor and vaginal delivery. The baby was in a right occipitoposterior presentation. (From Carreiro 2003.)

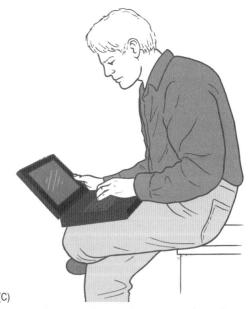

(C)

Figure 2.1C   Postural stress relating to casual use of laptop computer. Note in particular head, shoulder and spinal strain.

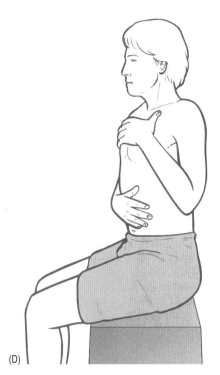

(D)

Figure 2.1D   Observation assessment of respiratory function. Any tendency for the upper hand to move cephalad, or earlier than the caudad hand, suggests scalene overactivity. (From Chaitow 2001.)

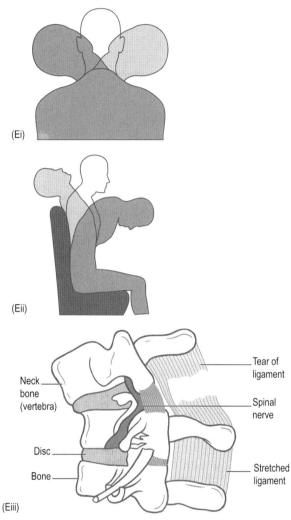

(Ei)

(Eii)

(Eiii)

Figure 2.1E   Patterns of whiplash stress relating to rear-end and side impacts.

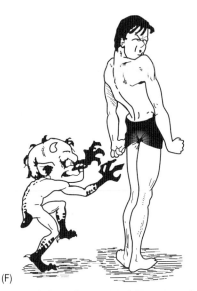

(F)

Figure 2.1F   Latey's lower fist, posterior. (From *Journal of Bodywork and Movement Therapies* 1(1): 49 with thanks to the artist Maxwell John Phipps.)

areas of dysfunction and embryonic triggers. When considering the effects on function and pain of reflex problems such as trigger points we need to remember that these were themselves caused by something else, so the detective work needs to look beyond the obvious. A trigger point that is causing pain in the back was itself caused by one or other, or a combination, of the features in this list, and simply 'deactivating' it (see Chapter 7) is not enough.

Chronic somatization influences, in which negative psychological factors and emotional coping tendencies, such as chronic fear, anger, anxiety or depression, will encourage musculoskeletal changes, including development of trigger points. Even though most manual therapists are not trained in psychotherapy it is important to at least understand the possibility of links between muscle and joint pain and chronic emotional states (see Box 2.1, and Fig. 2.1F).

A variety of *biochemical* imbalances can contribute to trigger point development (see Box 2.2). As with psychological influences, most manual therapists are

---

Box 2.1   Psychosocial influences on myofascial pain problems

When negative emotions (fear, hatred, anxiety, etc.) exist for lengthy periods, changes take place in the soft tissues that can lead to pain, restriction and the evolution of trigger points.

One way that this happens has been described by research (Waersted et al 1992, 1993).

It seems that the effect of psychological influences on muscles is more complicated than a simplistic 'whole muscle' or region being involved.

Researchers showed that a small number of muscle fibers, in particular muscles, display almost constant or repeated activity when a person is psychologically stressed.

The researchers tested the effects on the trapezius muscle of a normal individual performing complicated mental arithmetic.

They reported:

In spite of low total activity level of the muscle, a small pool of low-threshold motor units may be under considerable load for prolonged periods of time. ... If tension provoking factors are frequently present, and the subject repeatedly recruits the same motor units, overload may follow, possibly resulting in a metabolic crisis and the appearance of Type 1 [postural] fibres with abnormally large diameters, or 'ragged-red' fibres, which are interpreted as a sign of mitochondrial overload.

This is a description of the birth of a trigger point, involving an 'energy/metabolic crisis' – as described later in this chapter (Mense & Simons 1992).

This research is important because it strongly suggests that emotional stress can selectively involve postural fibers of muscles, which as described earlier, shorten over time when stressed. (see Box 2.7 on muscle types).

Just how localized the focus of stress can be is illustrated by two research studies conducted in the 1990s in California.

1. Needles were placed in myofascial trigger points located in the upper trapezius muscles of 14 individuals, in order to measure electrical activity (McNulty et al 1994). At the same time needles were also placed in non-trigger point fibers of the upper trapezius muscle. The people being tested were then asked to perform difficult mental arithmetic. There was immediate increase in electrical muscle activity *in the trigger points* when there was emotional stress, but not in the adjacent muscle tissues, which remained electrically silent. These results suggest a mechanism by which emotional factors directly influence muscle pain via areas that have become facilitated.

2. Needles were placed in trigger points (within 2 millimeters of the nodule in the taut band) and also in non-tender adjacent muscle tissue in people with

Box 2.1   Psychosocial influences on myofascial pain problems – *cont'd*

muscular pain and headache, as well as in people with no symptoms (Hubbard & Berkoff 1993). There was sustained spontaneous electromyographic activity in trigger points in the patients with pain, but no activity in people without symptoms. This suggests that trigger points are strongly influenced by increased sympathetic activity (see Box 2.3).

Somatization

Sometimes musculoskeletal symptoms may represent an unconscious attempt by the person to 'bury' their emotional distress.

The person may be somatizing this distress, and developing what seem to be purely biomechanical problems.

Lewit (1999) suggests that if a patient is able to give a fairly *precise* description and localization of his pain, we should not think of this as 'merely psychological' – there is likely to be a very real physical situation that needs investigating.

He also suggests that it is probable that vague pain symptoms, which are both hard to describe and hard to precisely locate, have a large psychological component.

Lewit notes that:

> The most important symptom [associated with psychological distress] is disturbed sleep. Characteristically, the patient falls asleep normally but wakes within a few hours and cannot get back to sleep.

The patient's history might provide clues about major psychological involvement, especially if this is a 'thick file' individual, someone who has consulted many people before you.

In masked depression, Lewit (1999) says the reported symptoms may be of vertebral pain, particularly involving the cervical region, with associated muscle tension and 'cramped' posture.

Becker (1991) informs us that people who somatize ('locking' their emotions into their physical structures) may go for years without an adequate diagnosis, often with misdiagnosis:

> Certain individuals, emotionally shortchanged or scarred during their formative years, show a [tendency] to somatize in the face of stressful events and circumstances of adult life, especially ones that awaken feelings buried in the unconscious and rooted in the past.

How are you to recognize such a patient?

According to Becker, when taking the history, look for:

- a vague and hard-to-believe history
- symptoms that proliferate and link different body areas
- highly emotionally charged descriptions (e.g. pain that is *searing*, *blinding*, *cruel*, etc.)
- exaggeration ('I couldn't move')
- discrepancies (e.g. the patient reports 'I cannot sit', but sits for the duration of the interview)
- passivity (e.g. resigned acceptance of disabled status)
- evidence of deconditioning, weight gain and/or increased use of narcotic medication.

Other signs might include the following:

- Tearfulness during the interview.
- Denial of a possible link between symptoms and emotional status. Many people feel threatened that they will be labeled as neurotic; or will be told, 'It's all in your mind', and seem to actively resent any link being suggested between their symptoms and their emotional state. This is a very delicate area and requires great tact.
- Anger directed at employer or doctors may be a displaced anger at the patient's parents.
- Failure of reasonable treatments – the patient may report worsening symptoms to the confusion of the practitioner because nothing aggravating has been done.
- Practitioner (you) may start feeling anger towards the patient (a process known as counter-transference).
- 'Emotional hunger' may be masked by increased weight gain, and excessive use of pain-relieving medication.

Caution

Despite the importance of the warnings suggested by Becker and others, it is important to remember that a great many people with widespread pain, and virtual disability, have very real musculoskeletal (or associated) conditions, and that their psychological distress may be a direct *result* of the pain and disability they are suffering, and not the cause.

The truth is that we should avoid splitting 'mind' from the 'body' when considering the source of pain. What is certain is that psychological distress can help to create trigger points.

Box 2.2   Biochemical aggravating and perpetuating factors of myofascial trigger points

Biochemical changes resulting from nutritional, toxic, endocrine, infectious and other influences can all encourage formation of trigger points, or help to perpetuate them (Simons et al 1999) (see Chapter 4).

Among the most important deficiencies identified as being associated with trigger points are:

vitamin B12 – deficiency is often linked to tiredness and specific neurological signs
folic acid – deficiency is associated with loose bowel movements, and also with feelings of coldness
vitamin C
iron – Simons et al (1999) report that about 10 to 15% of people with chronic myofascial pain problems are iron deficient. The patient is also likely to report feeling very cold, and to be easily fatigued – something that also applies to thyroid hormone deficiency (see below).

Chronic viral, parasite and yeast *infections* (e.g. *Candida*) are also possible perpetuating factors (Ferguson & Gerwin 2004).

There is a great deal of evidence suggesting that hormonal imbalances, sometimes involving *estrogen deficiency* but more commonly *thyroid deficiency*, may be involved in myofascial pain problems (Lowe & Honeyman-Lowe 1998). See Chapter 9 for more on this topic.

Thyroid imbalance is also associated with symptoms such as hair loss, roughened skin, feelings of coldness, extreme fatigue, weight gain and a tendency to constipation.

Allergic and sensitivity reactions have also been shown to be capable of having a strong influence on myofascial pain (Brostoff 1992).

---

not trained as nutritional experts. Nevertheless a basic understanding of what constitutes a balanced diet, and details of the patient's eating and drinking habits, might alert you to necessary changes. Although specific advice may not be appropriate (or legal if your license does not allow this), it is perfectly appropriate to pass on printed information, or to refer the person to a colleague for nutritional advice.

Once sensitized, an active trigger point (or facilitated spinal segment) can be irritated by any stressor, ranging from *psychological* or emotional stress that increases sympathetic arousal, or by physical, chemical, or *climatic* factors (e.g. humidity, extreme heat or cold, weather change, etc.) (Guedj & Weinberger 1990) (see Box 2.3).

What's actually happening in a trigger point?

Until recently the answer to this question would have been based on theory.

Now, thanks to some remarkable research at the National Institutes for Health it is possible to say precisely what happens at the heart of a trigger point, even if the theories as to why it happens remain unproven (Shah et al 2003).

The research methods are described in Box 2.4.

Progression from acute to chronic dysfunction

The first time you play tennis, dig the garden, paint a ceiling or perform any unaccustomed task, the muscles that are doing the work will be sore afterwards.

You will not be surprised, and you will know that unless you have actually injured yourself the soreness will vanish in a day or so (helped by some massage, and possibly hydrotherapy, to speed up the circulation and drainage of the area).

If you repeat the same activity regularly there will no longer be soreness afterwards, and slowly but surely the muscles doing the work will get used to it, and will probably get stronger.

We call this training, or more accurately adaptation, and even more accurately specific adaptation to imposed demand (SAID).

Take, for example, the specific adaptation of a weight-lifter, who would be very well tuned to lifting weights, but who would find it difficult to perform a high jump.

Also consider the wonderfully integrated activities of a gymnast whose performance demands coordination that can only be achieved by ensuring that training includes activities that coordinate strength, stamina, flexibility, stability and balance (Fig. 2.2, p. 27).

The first few sessions of almost any form of training will produce an alarm (acute) response, involving soreness and mild inflammation.

By repeating the SAID/training the changes will become chronic.

Examples are illustrated in Figure 2.3 (p. 27), where the particular muscles that are likely to be overused and stressed in a golfer (A) and a javelin thrower (B) are shown.

Adaptation of this sort involves changes – over time – that may be useful for the particular regular

Box 2.3   The sympathetic-parasympathetic nervous systems (Butler & Moseby 2003, Mense & Simons 2001)

Our lives are protected by the ability of the sympathetic nervous system to rapidly create a situation where we can defend ourselves or flee ('fight or flight'), and by the parasympathetic nervous system's ability to restore a calming balance.

Of course the story is more complicated than this, and involves coordinated hormonal release involving the pituitary, hypothalamus and adrenal glands.

The alarm rings, or a wild animal attacks, and we are instantly prepared to run, or to fight.

The sense of alarm itself derives from messages reaching the brain from the hundreds of thousands of sensors, those in the muscles, joints and fascia (proprioceptors, nociceptors, thermoreceptors, mechanoreceptors, etc.), as well as those in the eyes and ears.

All these messages are filtered through the brain, which has been programmed by its memories of past experiences ('This was painful last time, it will be the same or worse this time'), thoughts ('This is dangerous'), and beliefs ('Hurt means harm'), as well as by its present state of vulnerability (How many other stress burdens are being coped with? What is the present level of background anxiety?).

The hypothalamus and the pituitary gland in the brain send chemical messages to the adrenal glands (above the kidneys) so that, at the moment of alarm, epinephrine (adrenaline) and cortisol are poured into the system.

These vital hormones are protective, and possibly life-saving, in alarm settings such as this.

Interestingly one of the defining features of body-wide pain syndrome, fibromyalgia, is that cortisol levels are very low, showing a poor hormonal ability to cope with stress (Ferraccioli et al 1990).

This coincides with the sympathetic nervous system becoming increasingly active to prepare to carry out the fight-or-flight activities – the pupils dilate, salivary glands and digestive functions shut down, heart rate and blood pressure increase, muscles tense and prepare for action.

Interestingly, other features of fibromyalgia are the low levels of sympathetic and parasympathetic activity (Martinez-Lavin 1998).

When normal epinephrine (adrenaline) release occurs, and sympathetic arousal takes place, in response to stress, already sensitized (facilitated) areas such as trigger points will feel much more painful.

In a short-lived alarm situation epinephrine (adrenaline) will be released and sympathetic activity will increase – leading to a rapid response to the threat.

When the danger passes, parasympathetic calming influences start to operate, reducing epinephrine (adrenaline) and cortisol levels to normal.

If all this happens as described, no harm will have been done.

But what would happen if someone was frequently sympathetically aroused?

And what would happen if epinephrine (adrenaline) and cortisol (both of which are vital and useful in the short term, but harmful if too frequently present) were repeatedly released?

This is precisely what happens in a stressful life, where there may be home discord, problems in relationships, a demanding work environment, economic worries, deadlines to meet, never enough time, exams or interviews to prepare for, inadequate sleep or exercise, and all too commonly an unbalanced diet containing stimulants such as caffeine, alcohol and nicotine (all of which stimulate the adrenal glands and increase sympathetic activity).

This is a formula for reduced healing potential, memory decline, and possibly depression – along with increased pain and exhaustion, accompanied by trigger point activity.

As we can see in the reports in Box 2.1, on the effect of increased moderate stress (mental arithmetic, or pain), sympathetic arousal also has direct effects on trigger point activity.

---

task, but which may be physiologically undesirable for other tasks.

The overdevelopment of particular muscles will inevitably result in imbalance between the overactive muscles, and their inhibited antagonists (described further later in this chapter), and trigger points are likely to be a part of the adaptation process.

If the activities that are repeated are actually stressful, strain will result, and trigger points will almost certainly develop (Figs 2.4 and 2.5, p. 28).

It is not difficult to see that an area of the body that is painful, or distressed, may be progressing from acute to chronic dysfunction in overused and stressed muscles, whether the activity is weight training, postural stress, performing a massage, sitting at a computer, or any other activity (together with possible nutritional and/or

---

Box 2.4   What's happening at the heart of a trigger point?

In a study by Shah et al (2003), a hollow acupuncture needle was created into which two tiny tubes were inserted. Each tube was connected to a machine so that saline (salt) solution could be pumped through one, while the other was capable of sucking fluid from the tissues into which the needle was inserted. This process is described as microdialysis.

The fluids could then be carefully analyzed.

- Nine people were selected for the study.
- Three had neck pain and active trigger points in their upper trapezius muscles.
- Three had no neck pain, but had latent trigger points in the same muscle.
- Three others had no neck pain and no trigger points.

A pressure algometer was used (see Chapter 7) to record how much pressure was needed to produce pain when the trigger points were pressed (the pain threshold).

Using ultrasound imaging, the hollow needle was moved, in very small stages, toward the heart of a trigger point (its taut band) until it touched the bands of the six people whose trigger points (three active, three latent) had been identified by palpation.

At each small stage of the needle's penetration of the tissues, samples were taken of the fluid.

The same region of upper trapezius was penetrated by the needle, and samples taken, in the three people without trigger points, to compare the nature of the fluids extracted.

In this way multiple samples, from the three groups, were obtained and could be compared.

The most important findings were:

- The people with active points had a very much lower pain threshold than the other people studied, showing that the points were more irritable.
- The people with active points had much higher levels of substances such as bradykinin, norepinephrine (noradrenaline), interleukin-1 and substance P than the people with latent, or no, trigger points. (See Chapter 1 for the importance of these substances in creating sensitization of tissues).
- The level of acidity (pH) of the tissues in the region of the trigger point was very much greater (i.e. there was lower pH) than the others tested.

In a personal communication, the lead researcher has mentioned that the pH returned to normal almost instantly when the taut band was released, when the needle touched it, as did levels of oxygen.

---

emotional stresses) that asks the soft tissues of the body to adapt repetitively or constantly (Fig. 2.6, p. 29).

An adaptation sequence

The following features are commonly involved, and it is during such a sequence that trigger points often develop.

- An initial sympathetic 'alarm' response will occur in which tissues become hypertonic.
- If this continues for more than a brief period, oxygen levels in the muscle will drop (the reasons for, and effects of, this are explained in Box 2.5, p. 30).
- When oxygen levels are low, energy production (ATP) switches to what is known as *anaerobic glycolysis* (cellular production of energy without oxygen).
- This leads to the production of waste products such as lactic and pyruvic acid (Pryor & Prasad 2002).
- If circulation and drainage are reduced, because of the increased hypertonicity, these irritant substances cause discomfort or pain.

- Discomfort and/or pain increases hypertonicity even more, and irritates the local nerve receptors that report pain (nociceptors), and these become increasingly sensitized and facilitated (Korr 1978). (See sensitization discussion in Chapter 1, and Fig. 1.2.)
- Processes begin that (unless stopped) lead to cross-linkage and shortening of tissues, which gradually, over a period of months and years, become more fibrous and indurated (Fig. 2.7, p. 29).
- Changes occur in the way the body manufactures protein (protein synthesis), reducing the efficiency of tissue repair and regeneration.
- Trigger points evolve – see later in this chapter and in Chapter 3 for more detailed descriptions of how this happens (and Box 2.4 for the chemical processes at the heart of the trigger point).
- Tendons that are associated with tense muscles become overloaded and painful.
- Sustained tension in muscles leads to constant pulling on the tendinous attachments to bone (the

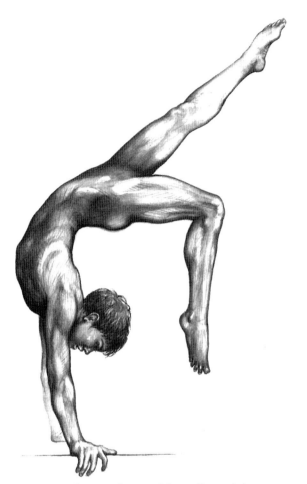

Figure 2.2   The miraculous possibilities of human balance. (From *Gray's Anatomy*, 38th edn.)

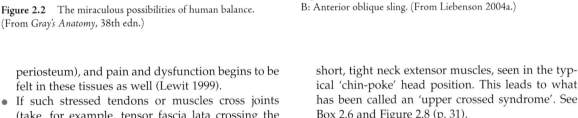

Figure 2.3   Oblique muscle slings: A: Posterior oblique sling. B: Anterior oblique sling. (From Liebenson 2004a.)

periosteum), and pain and dysfunction begins to be felt in these tissues as well (Lewit 1999).

- If such stressed tendons or muscles cross joints (take, for example, tensor fascia lata crossing the hip joint), these become crowded, and their function may be modified.
- The antagonists of chronically tense muscles will be weakened (reciprocally inhibited) and, as a result, normal firing sequences of muscles may change (Janda 1996).
- An example of this involves short, tight, erector spinae muscles and their weakened (inhibited) antagonists, the abdominal muscles, as seen in the typical slouching, pot-bellied, swayback, posture. This leads to what has been called a 'lower crossed syndrome'. See Box 2.6 and Figure 2.9 (p. 31).
- Another example would be the inhibition of deep neck flexor muscles because of the influence of

short, tight neck extensor muscles, seen in the typical 'chin-poke' head position. This leads to what has been called an 'upper crossed syndrome'. See Box 2.6 and Figure 2.8 (p. 31).

- Both these 'crossed patterns' make normal breathing difficult, encouraging upper chest patterns (see later in this chapter for more on this important topic).
- To prove this to yourself, stand tall and breathe deeply. Then slump, let your belly hang forward and your chin poke out. Now try to take a deep breath!
- This pattern of breathing puts a lot of strain on the accessory breathing muscles (upper trapezius, serratus anterior, levator scapulae, sternomastoid, scalenes), leading to soft tissue changes in these, including trigger points. This sequence is described in more detail below.

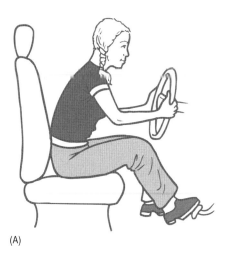

(A)

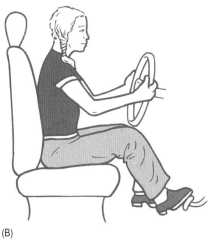

(B)

Figure 2.4   Driving: A: incorrect; B: correct. (From Liebenson 2004b.)

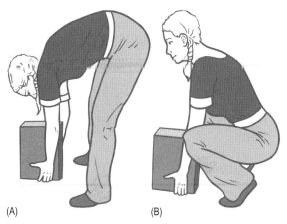

(A)   (B)

Figure 2.5   Lifting: A: incorrect; B: correct. (From Liebenson 2004b.)

they refer (see Fig. 2.11, p. 34, and the discussion of this later in this chapter – and in Chapter 1).

- Postural and functional changes will become apparent throughout the body, e.g. in relation to breathing pattern dysfunction ('upper chest breathing'), which becomes habitual and which can result from (for example) poor, slumped posture.
- Breathing pattern disorders cannot be easily normalized until the structural changes (short, tight muscles, for example) that are associated with them are corrected.

Unbalanced breathing and trigger points

Garland (1994) describes a series of muscular and joint changes (adaptations) that occur with chronic upper chest breathing:

- An imbalance develops between weak abdominal muscles and tight erector spinae muscles.
- Pelvic floor weakness develops.
- The upper ribs become elevated and there will be tension (and probably trigger points) in the intercostal muscles between the ribs.
- The thoracic spine becomes restricted because of poor rib movement.
- The scalenes, upper trapezius and levator scapulae all become hypertonic (and will eventually become fibrotic and develop trigger points).
- The cervical spine stiffens and may be painful.
- The tone of the diaphragm and core stabilizing muscles, such as transversus abdominus, will be affected (Hodges et al 2001, McGill et al 1995).

Overbreathing also causes what is known as respiratory alkalosis, because too much carbon

- In response to these postural and breathing pattern changes, chain reactions of dysfunction occur, involving the shortening – over time – of postural muscles (type 1 fibers), and the inhibition and weakening (without shortening) of phasic muscles (type 2 fibers) (see Box 2.7, p. 32).
- Localized areas of hyperreactivity (facilitation) may evolve in muscles alongside the spine, or in particular stress-prone regions of any myofascial structures – the beginning of trigger point development. (See the comparison of facilitation to a neurological 'lens', or to a sound system that has been turned up high, in Chapter 1.)
- In time trigger points themselves become sources of pain, and of further dysfunction, as embryonic (satellite) triggers develop in the areas to which

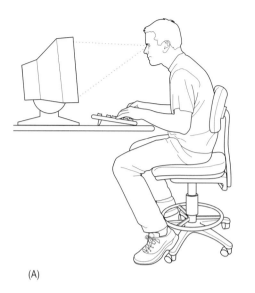

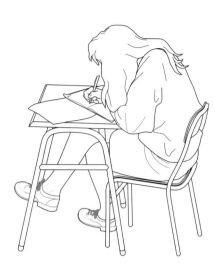

Figure 2.6   A: Inappropriate seated position for computer work forces head forward and stresses spine. B: Writing at a flat table of inappropriate height encourages distorted posture. (From Chaitow & DeLany

(A)   (B)

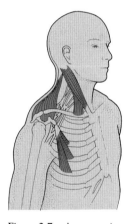
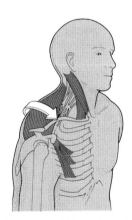

Figure 2.7   A progressive pattern of postural and biomechanical dysfunction develops, resulting in, and aggravated by, inappropriate breathing function. (From Chaitow 2001.)

dioxide is being exhaled (Chaitow et al 2002). When this happens blood vessels get narrower because of smooth muscle constriction, and the muscles, organs and brain receive less oxygen than they need to function normally. The tissues become ischemic and this encourages trigger points to develop (Mogyoros et al 1997, Seyal et al 1998). This is far more likely to happen in people who are out of condition and do not perform any aerobic exercise (Nixon & Andrews 1996).

These adaptation sequences inevitably lead to physiologically unsustainable adaptive changes, which lead to chronic myofascial and joint problems, almost inevitably including trigger point development.

Figure 2.11 (p. 34) shows a selection of trigger point locations and their referral, or radiating, target areas (zones of influence).

Chapter 4 contains a comprehensive series of 'maps' that should help direct you to the muscles in which active trigger points responsible for the pain are likely to be located.

This selection of trigger point sites, in named muscles, and their referral zones, should be seen as an important resource when you are attempting to link a patient's reported pain with possible trigger point influence.

Therapeutic choices

The treatment of the symptoms of pain and restriction, as a result of this progression from acute to chronic musculoskeletal adaptation, can be simplified into three broad categories: improving function, reducing the adaptive load and treatment of symptoms.

A full assessment should be made involving trying to discover:
What's too tight?
What's too loose?
What hurts?
What makes the pain worse, and what makes it better?
What's happening in these tissues, in this person at this time? ... and why?
How acute or chronic is the situation?

The answers to these questions help to decide what treatment choices are safe to introduce, based on the following broad treatment objectives.

1. Improving function
This might include use of methods that improve circulation and drainage; enhance posture; rehabilitate

Box 2.5   Ischemia and trigger point evolution

Ischemia can be described as a state in which the current oxygen supply is not adequate for the current physiological needs of the tissues.

Hypoxia involves tissues being deprived of adequate oxygen, and can occur in a number of ways.

- For example, circulation may be reduced due to tense muscles, resulting from overuse or overstrain.
- There are also areas where there is only limited blood supply at the best of times (known as hypovascularity), for example the area close to the insertion of the infraspinatus tendon, and the intercapsular aspect of the biceps tendon (Tullos & Bennet 1984).
- When tissues have to endure prolonged compression crowding, such as when side-lying during sleep, ischemia may occur under the acromion process (Brewer 1979).
- This can produce pain as well as spasm, vasoconstriction, weakness, loss of coordination and loss of work tolerance in the muscles of the area (Simons et al 1999).
- These are of course precisely the sites most associated with rotator cuff tendinitis, calcification and spontaneous rupture, as well as trigger point activity (Cailliet 1991).

Pain receptors (nociceptors) are sensitized when under ischemic conditions, due to bradykinin (a chemical mediator of inflammation) influence (Digiesi et al 1975).

When ischemia ceases, the sensitized pain receptor remains in this distressed state, and this assists in the creation of myofascial trigger points (Kieschke et al 1988).

As we have seen earlier in this chapter, ischemia occurs in trigger points as a result of the sequence of events that leads to excess calcium release and decreased ATP (energy) production.

Trigger point activity also encourages relative ischemia in 'target' tissues (Baldry 1993).

According to Simons et al (1999), these *target zones* (where pain is felt) are usually peripheral to the trigger point, sometimes central to the trigger point, and more rarely (27% of the time), the trigger point is located within the target zone of referral.

This means that if you are treating only the area of reported pain, and the cause is myofascial trigger points activity, you are 'in the wrong spot' nearly 75% of the time!

breathing; loosen and stretch whatever has tightened; increase tone and strength in whatever has weakened (or that has been inhibited); improve stamina; mobilize joints; deactivate trigger points – all with an objective of a long-term achievement of optimum flexibility, mobility, stability and balance, and an ability to better handle the demands of life.

A major part of this aspect of care would probably involve a variety of manual/massage methods including trigger point deactivation (see Chapters 7, 8 and 9).

2. Reducing the adaptive load

This may include – as far as is possible – methods that help the patient to modify work and leisure activities, and to change and improve habitual patterns of use; encourage more exercise; learn stress coping and relaxation methods; improve diet and lifestyle patterns – all with an objective of lowering the number and intensity of compensation and adaptation demands being placed on the soft and hard tissues of the body, whether these are of biomechanical, biochemical or psychosocial origin. The approaches required include education, instruction and home-work.

3. Treatment of symptoms

This would include use of treatment methods that ease pain, relax tension and improve function in the short term, as far as this is possible, as the longer-term changes, outlined above, are taking place. A part of these treatment approaches should involve massage and trigger point deactivation.

But it is important to keep in mind that simply taking a hammer to smash a fire alarm will not do anything about the reason that the alarm is ringing! Deactivating a trigger point, without paying attention to why it exists, would be about as sensible as this example.

THE SMALL PICTURE

As the large adaptive influences described above impact on the body, changes are taking place in the tissues of the body right down to the cellular level.

Mense & Simons (2001) have described what is thought to happen to create a trigger point, based on the research of Simons et al (1999) (Fig. 2.12, p. 35).

- Microtrauma (caused by overuse, misuse, abuse – see above) to part of a muscle spindle, the sarcoplasmic reticulum (which wraps around each muscle fibril), causes acetylcholine (ACh) to be released, and this in turn results in release of calcium stored in the muscle cells.

Box 2.6   Crossed syndrome patterns

Among the commonest body-wide stress influences are postural patterns such as the upper and lower crossed syndromes (Janda 1996).

Upper crossed syndrome pattern

The upper crossed syndrome involves a round-shouldered, chin-poking, slumped, posture that crowds the thorax and prevents normal breathing (Fig. 2.8).

The chest, neck, shoulder and thoracic spine are all likely to be sites of pain and restriction as a result.

The associated muscles, most particularly upper trapezius, levator scapulae, pectoralis major and minor, sternomastoid as well as most of the cervical and spinal muscles of the upper back, will either shorten, or weaken and lengthen (particularly deep neck flexor muscles), depending on their classification as postural or phasic (see Box 2.7).

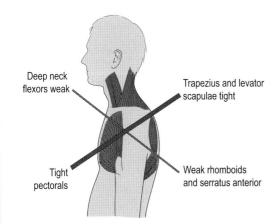

Deep neck flexors weak

Trapezius and levator scapulae tight

Tight pectorals

Weak rhomboids and serratus anterior

Figure 2.8   The upper crossed syndrome, as described by Janda. (From Chaitow 2001.)

Lower crossed syndrome pattern

The lower crossed syndrome involves a typical 'sway-back' posture with slack abdominal and gluteal muscles, and over-tight erector spinae, quadratus lumborum, tensor fascia lata, piriformis and psoas (Fig. 2.9).

Trigger points are found in abundance in both postural and phasic muscles, but more abundantly in postural ones.

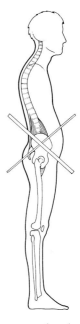

Figure 2.9   The lower crossed syndrome, as described by Janda. (From Chaitow 2001.)

- Microtrauma has been observed in relation to repetitive strain injuries, high-velocity injuries such as occur in athletics or motor accidents, and postural or occupationally stressful postures (Kostopoulos & Rizopoulos 2001).
- This calcium release causes myosin and actin filaments to slide, shortening the sarcomere, and producing a local contracture (a taut band) (Fig. 2.13, p. 35).
- The shortening of the sarcomeres creates a 'knot' or nodule. This is often palpable when searching for trigger points (Fig. 2.14, p. 35).
- The taut band can also usually be palpated, unless the trigger point is lying in very deep muscle.
- It is important to remember that this muscle fiber contracture is not controlled by nerve activity (motor potential), but happens because of the chemical imbalance (involving the excessive release of ACh and calcium, as described above).
- This process demands a great deal of oxygen, which cannot be supplied in sufficient quantities because of the contracture.
- This leads to what is known as hypoxia – oxygen levels below what the tissues need to function normally.
- Because of the microtrauma there is also likely to be a release of chemical irritants, such as bradykinin.
- All this produces some protective muscle guarding, as well as local swelling (edema) that compresses the tiny blood vessels that carry oxygen and remove waste products.

Box 2.7   Different muscle types: postural (type 1) and phasic (type 2)

Janda (1986) and Lewit (1999) state that there are two basic muscle activities and types:

Type 1 – those muscles whose functions are mainly postural tend to shorten and become hypertonic when stressed, abused, or under- or overused.

Type 2 – those muscles whose functions are mainly phasic tend to hypotonia, weakening and atrophy under conditions of under- or overuse, or abuse.

All muscles contain both type 1 and type 2 fibers. The muscles' type – postural or phasic – depends on which of the fiber types is greatest.

There are other classification methods used to describe different muscle types and functions. In some the muscles are divided into 'stabilizers' and 'mobilizers'; in others they are described as 'global' and 'local'. In this book the descriptors used by Janda and Lewit have been chosen (postural and phasic).

Postural muscles (Fig. 2.10) include :
- tibialis posterior
- gastrocnemius-soleus
- rectus femoris
- iliopsoas
- tensor fascia lata
- hamstrings
- short thigh adductors
- quadratus lumborum
- piriformis
- some paravertebral muscles
- pectoralis major (and perhaps minor)
- sternocleidomastoid
- upper trapezius
- levator scapulae
- flexors of the upper extremity.

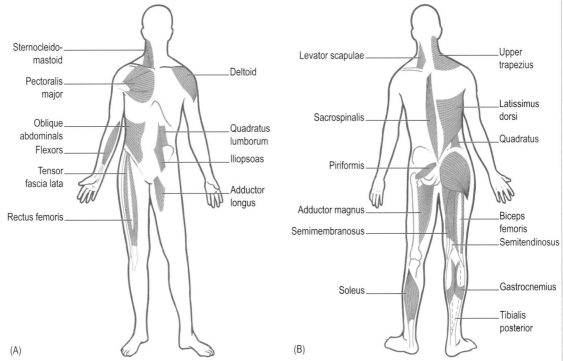

Figure 2.10   A: Major postural muscles of the anterior aspects of the body. B: Major postural muscles of the posterior aspects of the body. (From Chaitow 2003.)

Box 2.7   Different muscle types: postural (type 1) and phasic (type 2) – *cont'd*

A number of conditions exist in which specific patterns of dysfunction are associated with shortening of postural muscles (e.g. iliopsoas, piriformis, tensor fascia lata, and iliotibial band). These muscles are particularly prone to development of trigger points, although trigger points are also found in phasic muscles.

The *phasic muscles* include:
- tibialis anterior
- the vasti
- the glutei
- abdominal muscles (mainly the recti)

- lower stabilizers of the scapula
- some deep neck flexors
- extensors of the upper extremity.

Janda suggests that before any attempt is made to strengthen weakened muscles (using exercise), it is important for the shortened antagonists to be stretched and relaxed, removing inhibiting (weakening) influences.

If a start is made by exercising weakened phasic muscles this is likely to increase tone in the already tight antagonists.

- The pressure on the tiny blood vessels leads to ischemia (reduced blood supply) and even greater hypoxia (oxygen deficiency).
- Because of these processes energy production (ATP) drops, and there is not enough energy to switch off the ACh, or to clear the excess calcium, and this maintains the contracture in the muscle spindle.
- By this time there will be local tenderness, and local nerve structures (including the pain receptors) will have become irritated.
- A trigger point will have been created.
- As the trigger becomes more irritated it starts to radiate or refer pain.
- Embryonic trigger points will develop in the pain reference ('target') zone (Fig. 2.15, p. 36).
- The trigger point, therefore, is the result of an 'energy crisis' involving local irritation or trauma.

Wolfe & Simons (1992) describe the trigger point evolution as follows:

Visualize a spindle like a strand of yarn in a knitted sweater … a metabolic crisis takes place which increases the temperature locally in the trigger point, shortens a minute part of the muscle (sarcomere) – like a snag in a sweater – and reduces the supply of oxygen and nutrients into the trigger point. During this disturbed episode an influx of calcium occurs and the muscle spindle does not have enough energy to pump the calcium outside the cell where it belongs. Thus a vicious cycle is maintained; the muscle spindle can't seem to loosen up and the affected muscle can't relax.

There are a number of important trigger point features relating to where they are located. This aspect of understanding trigger points – and how it influences treatment choices – will be described in Chapter 3.

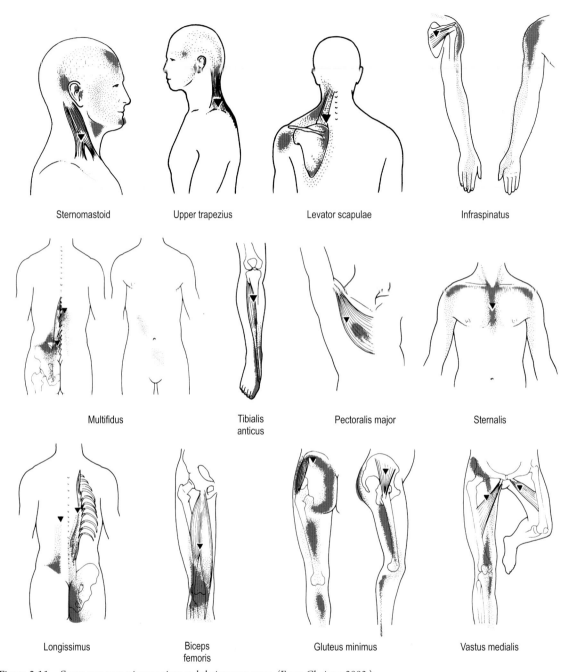

Sternomastoid   Upper trapezius   Levator scapulae   Infraspinatus

Multifidus   Tibialis anticus   Pectoralis major   Sternalis

Longissimus   Biceps femoris   Gluteus minimus   Vastus medialis

Figure 2.11 Some common trigger points and their target areas. (From Chaitow 2003.)

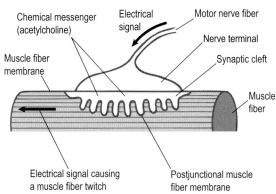

Figure 2.12 Motor endplate structure and function. Schematic cross-section shows how the electrical signal of the motor nerve is normally converted to a chemical signal and then back to an electrical signal. The original electrical signal causes the nerve terminal to simultaneously release many packets of acetylcholine that spread across the synapse. On arrival at the postjunctional membrane of the muscle cell, this chemical messenger is converted back to an electrical signal. Normally just a few packets per second of acetylcholine are released under resting conditions. (From Simons 2002.)

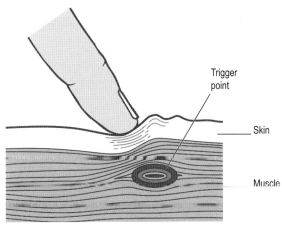

Figure 2.14 Trigger points are areas of local facilitation that can be housed in any soft tissue structure, most usually muscle and/or fascia. Palpation from the skin or at depth may be required to localize them. (From Chaitow 2003.)

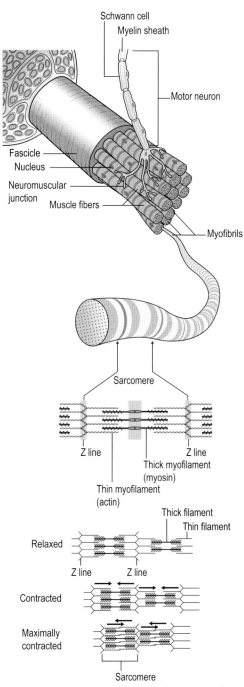

Figure 2.13 Each fascicle contains a bundle of muscle fibers. A group of fibers is innervated by a single motor neuron (each fiber individually at its neuromuscular junction). Each fiber consists of a bundle of myofibrils that are composed of sarcomeres laid end to end. The sarcomere contains the actin (thin) and myosin (thick) filaments, which serve as the basic contractile unit of skeletal muscles. (Adapted with permission from Thibodeau & Patton 2000.)

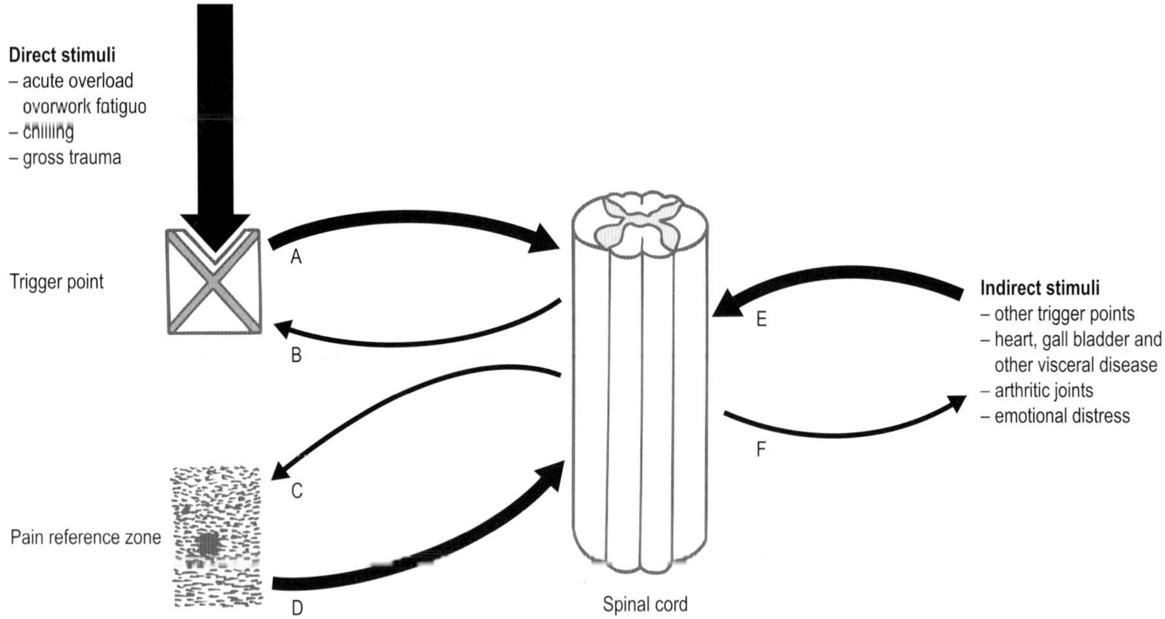

Direct stimuli
– acute overload
  overwork fatigue
– chilling
– gross trauma

Trigger point

A

B

Pain reference zone

C

D

E

F

Spinal cord

Indirect stimuli
– other trigger points
– heart, gall bladder and
  other visceral disease
– arthritic joints
– emotional distress

Figure 2.15   Direct stress influence can affect the hyperreactive neural structure of a myofascial trigger point, leading to increased activity (A–B) as well as referring sensations (pain, paresthesia, increased sympathetic activity) to a target area (C–D) that feed back into the cord to increase the background stress load. Other stimuli reach the cord from distant trigger points and additional dysfunctional areas (E–F). (From Chaitow 2003.)

CLINICAL NOTE

Key points from Chapter 2

1. Faced with numerous stress demands (overuse, poor posture, upper chest breathing, etc.), tissues modify in stages from acute to chronic adaptation.

2. In the process of adaptation ischemia is often a feature, as is the presence of irritant substances that sensitize tissues.

3. Increased sympathetic activity is another feature of early adaptive responses.

4. Muscles can be divided into different types (postural and phasic), and these behave differ-

ently in response to overuse and stress – postural muscles shorten, phasic muscles weaken.

5. Out of this background of general and local adaptation responses an energy crisis may occur in myofascial tissue, involving calcium release, local contracture, energy deficit, etc., and this allows the development of trigger points

6. These adaptive changes are more likely if there is also psychological/emotional stress, and/or biochemical imbalance (nutritional, hormonal, etc.).

References

Baldry P 1993 Acupuncture, trigger points and musculoskeletal pain. Churchill Livingstone, Edinburgh

Becker G 1991 Chronic pain. Depression and the injured worker. Psychiatric Annals 21(1):391–404

Brewer B 1979 Aging and the rotator cuff. American Journal of Sports Medicine 7:102–110

Brostoff J 1992 Complete guide to food allergy. Bloomsbury, London

Butler D, Moseby L 2003 Explain pain. Noigroup, Adelaide

Cailliet R 1991 Shoulder pain. F A Davis, Philadelphia

Carreiro J 2003 An osteopathic approach to children. Churchill Livingstone, Edinburgh p 119–120

Chaitow L 2001 Muscle energy techniques, 2nd edn. Churchill Livingstone, Edinburgh

Chaitow L 2003 Modern neuromuscular techniques, 2nd edn. Churchill Livingstone, Edinburgh

Chaitow L, DeLany J 2000 Clinical application of neuromuscular techniques. Vol 2, Lower body. Churchill Livingstone, Edinburgh

Chaitow L, Bradley D, Gilbert C 2002 Multidisciplinary approaches to breathing pattern disorders. Churchill Livingstone, Edinburgh

Digiesi V et al 1975 Effect of proteinase inhibitor on intermittent claudication. Pain 1:385–389

Ferguson L W, Gerwin R 2004 Clinical mastery of treatment of myofascial pain. Lippincott Williams & Wilkins, Philadelphia, p 22

Ferraccioli G, Cavalieri F, Salaffi F et al 1990 Neuroendocrinological findings in primary fibromyalgia and other rheumatic conditions. Journal of Rheumatology 17:869–873

Garland W 1994 Somatic changes in hyperventilating subject. Presentation at Respiratory Function Congress, Paris

Guedj D, Weinberger A 1990 Effect of weather conditions on rheumatic patients. Annals of the Rheumatic Diseases 49:158–159

Hodges P, Heinjnen I, Gandevia S 2001 Postural activity of the diaphragm is reduced in humans when respiratory demand increases. Journal of Physiology 537(3):999–1008

Hubbard D, Berkoff G 1993 Myofascial trigger points show spontaneous needle EMG activity. Spine 18(13):1803–1807

Janda V 1986 Muscle weakness and inhibition (pseudoparesis) in back pain syndromes. In: Grieve G (ed) Modern manual therapy of the vertebral column. Churchill Livingstone, Edinburgh

Janda V 1996 Evaluation of muscular imbalance. In: Liebenson C (ed) Rehabilitation of the spine. Williams & Wilkins, Baltimore

Kieschke J, Mense S, Prabhakar N R 1988 Influences of adrenaline and hypoxia on rat muscle receptors. Progress in Brain Research 74:91–97

Korr I 1978 Neurological mechanisms in manipulative therapy. Plenum Press, New York

Kostopoulos D Rizopoulos K 2001 The manual of trigger point and myofascial therapy. Slack Inc, Thorofare NJ, p 20

Lewit K 1999 Manipulation in rehabilitation of the motor system. Butterworth Heinemann, London

Liebenson C 2004a The relationship of the sacroiliac joint, stabilization musculature, and lumbo-pelvic instability. Journal of Bodywork and Movement Therapies 8(1):43–45

Liebenson C 2004b How to take care of your back. Journal of Bodywork and Movement Therapies 8(2):85–87

Lowe J, Honeyman-Lowe G 1998 Facilitating the decrease in fibromyalgic pain during metabolic rehabilitation. Journal of Bodywork and Movement Therapies 2(4):208–217

McGill S, Sharratt M, Seguin J 1995 Loads on spinal tissues during simultaneous lifting and ventilatory challenge. Ergonomics 38(9):1772–1792

McNulty W, Gevirtz R, Hubbard D 1994 Needle electromyographic evaluation of trigger point response to a psychological stressor Psychophysiology 31(3): 313–316

Martinez-Lavin M 1998 Circadian studies of autonomic nervous balance in patients with fibromyalgia. Arthritis and Rheumatism 41:1966–1971

Mense S Simons D 2001 Muscle pain. Lippincott Williams & Wilkins, Philadelphia

Mogyoros I, Kiernan K, Burke D et al 1997 Excitability changes in human sensory and motor axons during hyperventilation and ischaemia. Brain 120(2):317–325

Nixon P, Andrews J 1996 A study of anaerobic threshold in chronic fatigue syndrome (CFS). Biological Psychology 43(3):264

Pryor J, Prasad S 2002 Physiotherapy for respiratory and cardiac problems, 3rd edn. Churchill Livingstone, Edinburgh, p 81

Seyal M, Mull B, Gage B 1998 Increased excitability of the human corticospinal system with hyperventilation. Electroencephalography and Clinical Neurophysiology/Electromyography and Motor Control 109(3):263–267

Shah J, Phillips T, Danoff J, Gerber L 2003 A novel microanalytical technique for assaying soft tissue demonstrates significant quantitative biochemical differences in 3 clinically distinct groups: Normal, latent, and active. Archives of Physical Medicine 84:9

Simons D G 2002 Understanding effective treatments of myofascial trigger points. Journal of Bodywork and Movement Therapies 6(2):81–88

Simons D, Travell J, Simons L 1999 Myofascial pain and dysfunction: the trigger point manual, vol 1, 2nd edn. Williams & Wilkins, Baltimore

Thibodeau G, Patton K 2000 Structure and function of the body, 11th edn. Mosby, London

Tullos H, Bennet J 1984 The shoulder in sports. In: Scott W (ed) Principles of sports medicine. Williams & Wilkins, Baltimore

Waersted M, Eken T, Westgaard R 1992 Single motor unit activity in psychogenic trapezius muscle tension. Arbete och Halsa 17:319–321

Waersted M, Eken T, Westgaard R 1993 Psychogenic motor unit activity – a possible muscle injury mechanism studied in a healthy subject. Journal of Musculoskeletal Pain 1(3/4):185–190

Wolfe F, Simons D 1992 Fibromyalgia and myofascial pain syndromes. Journal of Rheumatology 19(6):944–995

CHAPTER THREE

Different trigger point characteristics

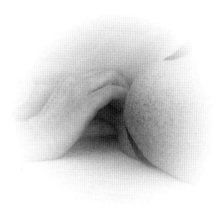

We have already seen that trigger points can be active or latent (see Box 1.1 in Chapter 1).

Those descriptions tell us how they behave.

Both active and latent trigger points produce pain when stimulated/pressed, but only an active point produces pain that the patient recognizes as being the same as their symptoms.

Whenever an active trigger point is identified (a painful, nodular point, lying in a taut band of soft tissue, with referral or radiating pain that is familiar to the patient) it is important to know whether this point lies near the center of a muscle, or close to one of its attachments.

Trigger points that are found in different parts of muscles have distinctive characteristics.

If a muscle has a trigger point close to its center (belly), it will usually also have trigger points at each of its attachments.

And similarly if a trigger point lies close to an attachment of a muscle (to its tendon or to bone) there will almost always be one near the center (belly) of the same muscle.

These 'central' and 'attachment' points need to be understood and treated quite differently, for very good reasons.

Where a point is located (central or attachment) decide whether it should be treated first, and also *how* it should be treated.

So, some triggers are active and others are latent; some triggers are near the center of a muscle and some are close to the attachment.

And some trigger points appear to be 'key' points (see Table 3.1).

This means that when a key point is deactivated, satellite points that are linked to it, in a virtual chain, will also be deactivated (or at least reduced in activity.)

Box 3.1 contains descriptions of the three main theories that try to explain how and why trigger points develop.

This partly repeats what has already been explained in Chapter 2.

By placing these three theories together in Box 3.1 you will have the chance to compare what is known (much of the description in this chapter) with what is thought to happen (as outlined in Chapter 2 in particular), in relation to trigger points.

CENTRAL AND ATTACHMENT POINTS

Simons et al (1999) have identified two locations where trigger points develop.

1. *Central trigger points* form close to the belly of the muscle (near the motor endpoint). It is important for manual therapists to become aware of the many different muscle shapes and locations. Once this has been achieved trigger point sites are fairly easy to predict. See Figures 3.2 and 3.3.

   Triggers develop following the sort of stresses and strains that occur in muscles (as described in previous chapters) and the sequence of local events listed in Chapter 2, that end in a 'crisis' involving acetylcholine (ACh) being released.

   As the endplate keeps producing a flow of ACh, a taut band and a 'knot' form, and as this process continues tension increases from the center, pulling on the ends of the muscle, the attachments. This starts to create the same sort of problems that will have taken place in the center, developing near the attachments. As this happens new trigger points form, adding to the general distress of the muscle, and local and referred pain.

Box 3.1   Theories of trigger point development

There are three main theories (and a number of minor ones) that attempt to explain just what is happening that allows a trigger point to evolve.

1. Energy crisis theory

This is the earliest explanation of trigger point formation (Bengtsson et al 1986, Hong 1996, Simons et al 1999).

The theory suggests that increased demand on a muscle, possibly involving repetitive, very small-grade trauma (microtrauma) or actual injury (macrotrauma), causes calcium release from muscle cells leading to shortening of the sarcomeres.

This has the effect of obstructing normal circulation, so that tissues receive less oxygen.

This causes the cells to be unable to produce enough energy (ATP) to allow the shortened sarcomeres to relax.

Waste products of metabolism accumulate (Simons et al 1999), and this causes some of the pain because of irritation and sensitization of sensory nerves (nociceptors).

This concept was partly supported by Bengtsson et al (1986).

2. The motor endplate theory

The motor nerve connects with a muscle cell at the motor endplate.

Research has shown that each trigger point contains very small areas (loci) that produce unusual electrical activity (Hubbard & Berkhoff 1993).

These loci are usually found at the motor endplate zone (Simons 2001, Simons et al 2002).

The activity seen on EMG (electromyogram) is thought to be the result of an increased rate of release of acetylcholine (ACh) from the nerve cell. This may be enough to cause activation of a few contractile elements and be responsible for some degree of muscle shortening (Simons 1996).

By combining these two theories (energy crisis and motor endplate), a basic model exists that helps explain the origin of the trigger point.

There is a third theory.

3. Radiculopathic model

Some researchers have a different model altogether. They think that there is a neurological cause, and that trigger points are a secondary phenomenon (Gunn 1997, Quintner & Cohen 1994).

Gunn (1997) suggests that myofascial pain often derives from intervertebral disc degeneration, which causes nerve root compression and paraspinal muscle spasm. This is described as a form of neuropathy (carpal tunnel syndrome is a neuropathy) that sensitizes and irritates structures in the distribution of the nerve root, and causes distal muscle spasm.

4. Polymodal theory (Fig. 3.1)

The polymodal receptor (PMR) hypothesis suggests that trigger points are nothing more than sensitized neural structures (pain receptors/nociceptors called polynodal receptors).

The PMR is a kind of nociceptor, and is responsive to mechanical acupuncture, thermal and chemical stimuli. Its sensory terminals are free nerve endings and exist in various tissues of the entire body. (Kawakita et al 2002)

Irrespective of which theory, or combination of theories, is actually proved to be correct, the fact remains that these noxious, painful trouble-makers cause a great deal of pain and dysfunction.

Box 3.1   Theories of trigger point development – *cont'd*

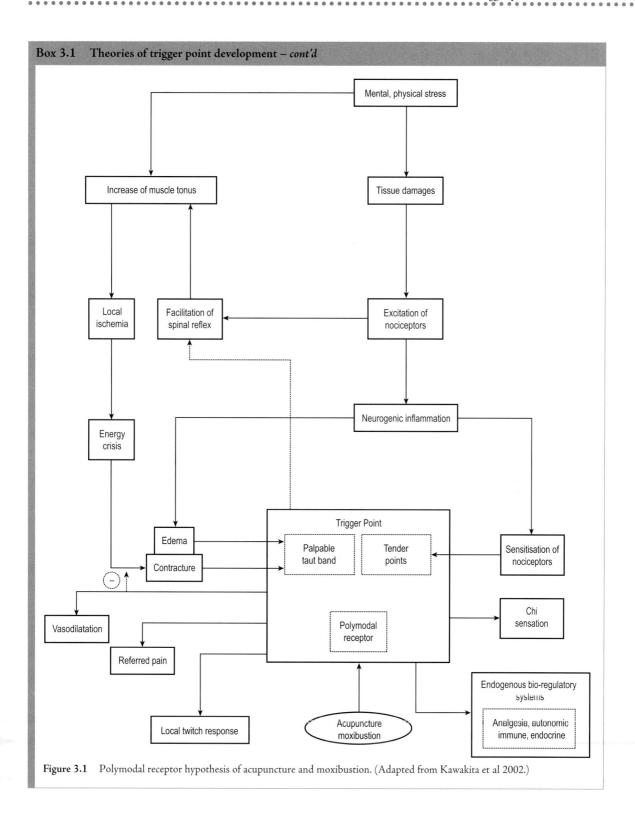

Figure 3.1   Polymodal receptor hypothesis of acupuncture and moxibustion. (Adapted from Kawakita et al 2002.)

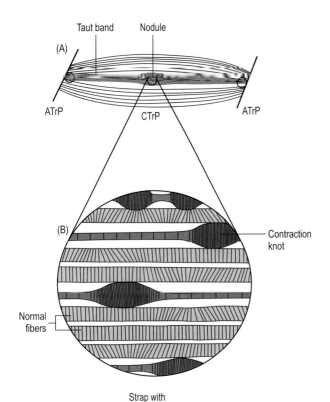

Figure 3.2 Tension produced by central trigger point can result in localized inflammatory response (attachment trigger point). (Adapted from Simons et al 1999.)

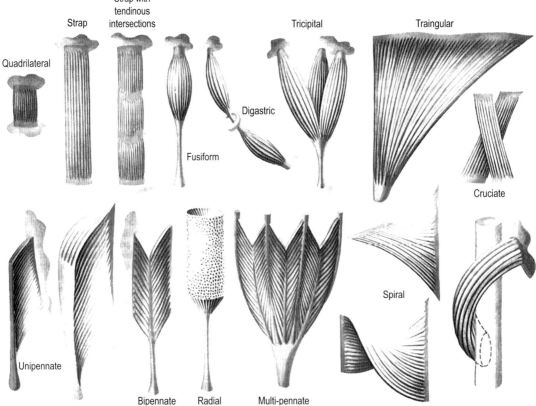

Figure 3.3 Types of muscle fiber arrangement. (From *Gray's Anatomy*, 38th edn.)

2. *Attachment trigger points* develop in the tissues where these shortened tissues merge with the tendons or bones associated with the muscle. Tension in these attachment tissues may lead not only to trigger points, but possibly to local inflammation, fibrosis and, eventually, deposition of calcium.

Different treatment methods for attachment and central trigger points

Simons and his colleagues have shown that both central and attachment trigger points can have the same end result – referred or radiating pain. However, the way these points develop is different, and the way they are treated should also be different.

- It is suggested that *attachment trigger points* should be treated by first releasing any associated central trigger point.
- And *central trigger points* should be treated while remembering that they involve contracted central sarcomeres, and local ischemia. See Box 2.5.
- When compression techniques are used in treatment of central trigger points, the oxygen supply changes because of the flush of blood through the tissues when the compression is released. This is even more likely if the pressure being applied is intermittent (on/off/on, etc., as described in Chapter 7).
- Central trigger points also usually respond well to heat applications (Kurz 1986).
- Because the tissues close to attachments can easily be irritated or inflamed (known as enthesopathy or enthesitis) it is important not to aggravate attachment trigger points by using deep pressure or friction.
- To prevent irritation of attachment areas only mild stretches should be used when treating central trigger points.
- Gliding (massage) techniques may usefully be applied, from the center of the fibers, out toward the attachments.
- By elongating the tissue toward the attachment in this way, shortened sarcomeres at the center of the muscle fiber will lengthen, and those that are over-stretched near the attachments will have the tension reduced.
- Because of the tendency toward inflammation, ice applications are more appropriate for attachment points, rather than heat. Short (20–30 seconds) cold applications cause a strong flushing of the tissues with fresh oxygen-rich blood, after the cold material is removed (Boyle & Saine 1988).

KEY AND SATELLITE TRIGGER POINTS

Research evidence suggests that 'key' triggers exist which, when deactivated, relieve activity in satellite trigger points (usually located within the target area of the key trigger).

If these key trigger points are not relieved, and only the satellites are treated, the referral pain pattern usually returns.

Hong & Simons (1992) have reported on over 100 trigger point sites that were inactivated by treatment of different (key) trigger points. Some of their findings are listed in Table 3.1.

Table 3.1   Key and satellite trigger points

Key trigger	Satellite trigger
Sternocleidomastoid	Temporalis, masseter, digastric
Upper trapezius	Temporalis, masseter, splenius, semispinalis, levator scapulae, rhomboid major
Scaleni	Deltoid, extensor carpi radialis, extensor digitorum communis, extensor carpi ulnaris
Splenius capitis	Temporalis, semispinalis
Supraspinatus	Deltoid, extensor carpi radialis
Infraspinatus	Biceps brachii
Pectoralis minor	Flexor carpi radialis, flexor carpi ulnaris, first dorsal interosseous
Latissimus dorsi	Triceps, flexor carpi ulnaris
Serratus posterior superior	Triceps, latissimus dorsi, extensor digitorum communis, extensor carpi ulnaris, flexor carpi ulnaris
Deep paraspinals	Gluteus maximus, medius and minimus, piriformis, hamstrings, tibialis, peroneus longus, gastrocnemius, soleus
Quadratus lumborum	Gluteus maximus, medius and minimus, piriformis
Piriformis	Hamstrings
Hamstrings	Peroneus longus, gastrocnemius, soleus

CLINICAL NOTE

Key points from Chapter 3

1. Some trigger points are active – the patient recognizes the symptoms (pain, etc.) as being 'familiar'.

2. Other trigger points are latent. The pain they produce is not familiar to the patient.

3. Latent points can nevertheless interfere with normal muscle function, and if sufficiently stressed can eventually become active.

4. When a trigger point is found it is important to decide whether it lies in the belly or close to the attachment of a muscle.

5. Triggers that form near the belly of the muscle (central points) require different therapeutic methods compared with attachment trigger points.

6. In general central points should be treated first.

7. Attachment points should be treated cautiously because inflammation is more likely in the tissues housing them, than it is in tissues housing central points.

8. Key trigger points can be identified which if deactivated will also reduce or eliminate activity in satellite points.

9. There are a number of theories (Box 3.1) that attempt to explain how and why trigger points develop. All the theories are partly supported by research.

References

Bengtsson A, Henrikkson K, Larsson J 1986 Reduced high energy phosphate levels in the painful muscles of patients with primary fibromyalgia. Arthritis and Rheumatism 29:817–821

Boyle W, Saine A 1988 Naturopathic hydrotherapy. Buckeye Naturopathic Press, East Palestine, OH

Gunn C 1997 Radiculopathic pain: diagnosis and treatment of segmental irritation or sensitisation. Journal of Musculoskeletal Pain 5:119–134

Hong C Z 1996 Pathophysiology of myofascial trigger point. Journal of the Formosan Medical Association 95(2):93–104

Hong C Z, Simons D 1992 Remote inactivation of myofascial trigger points by injection of trigger points in another muscle. Scandinavian Journal of Rheumatology 94(suppl):25

Hubbard D, Berkhoff G 1993 Myofascial trigger points show spontaneous needle EMG activity. Spine 18:1803–1807

Kawakita K, Itoh K, Okada K 2002 The polymodal receptor hypothesis of acupuncture and moxibustion, and its rational explanation of acupuncture points. International Congress Series: Acupuncture – is there a physiological basis? Elsevier Science, Amsterdam, 1238:63–68

Kurz I 1986 Textbook of Dr Vodder's manual lymph drainage, vol 2: therapy, 2nd edn. Karl F Haug, Heidelberg

Quintner J, Cohen M 1994 Referred pain of peripheral nerve origin: an alternative to the myofascial pain construct. Clinical Journal of Pain 10:243–251

Simons D 1996 Clinical and etiological update of myofascial pain from trigger points. Journal of Musculoskeletal Pain 4:93–121

Simons D 2001 Do endplate noise and spikes arise from normal motor endplates? American Journal of Physical Medicine and Rehabilitation 80:134–140

Simons D, Travell J, Simons L 1999 Myofascial pain and dysfunction: the trigger point manual, vol 1, 2nd edn. Williams & Wilkins, Baltimore

Simons D, Hong C-Z, Simons L 2002 Endplate potentials are common to midfiber myofascial trigger points. American Journal of Physical Medicine and Rehabilitation 81:212–222

CHAPTER FOUR

Maps and other ways of locating trigger points

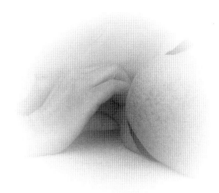

In this chapter, several different ways of identifying sources of pain that may *not* be caused by trigger points will be discussed, as will ways of identifying trigger points that may actually be causing painful symptoms.

1. The viscera (organs) can be a source of pain in muscles and joints, and it's important to be aware of this, so that the blame is not too quickly given to trigger points, when the real cause is something else altogether.
2. A variety of serious ailments can produce musculoskeletal symptoms that mimic trigger point pain. You need to be aware of these 'imposter' sources of pain.
3. Myofascial pain often arises from trigger points associated with scar tissue, and the importance of this will be emphasized.
4. Joint pain and restriction is often caused by trigger points. Maps will be presented that can help to identify which muscles might be the hosts to trigger points that are causing joint and soft tissue pain, in different parts of the body.
5. 'Key' trigger points influence satellite points that are usually distal (further from the head) to them. When a key trigger point is irritated satellite points also become more sensitive, and active in producing pain. Once a key trigger is deactivated, associated satellite points also switch off (see Table 3.1 in the previous chapter).
6. A selection of trigger points relating to headache and head/facial pain are illustrated toward the end of this chapter.

VISCERAL SOURCES OF PAIN

It is important to remember that muscular and joint pain can also derive from organ disease and dysfunction. See Figure 1.10.

● Viscerosomatic referrals (from organs to the musculoskeletal tissues – such as the arm pain often experienced with a heart attack) are also noted for other organs.
● Somatovisceral referrals (from musculoskeletal tissues to the organs) can be 'silent', because organs do not always report pain.
● However, repeated viscerosomatic referrals (such as low back pain that comes from a kidney stone, infection or disease) might be an organ's painful cry for help.

Figure 4.1 shows regions of the body that may become painful in response to heart or gallbladder or diaphragm disease or dysfunction.

Note that in this figure:

● D (diaphragm) refers to the trapezius area
● GB (gallbladder) refers to the shoulder and tip of the scapula on same side
● H (heart) refers to the chest wall and left arm (angina type pain).

Other visceral referral patterns

Figure 4.2 shows a variety of referral areas deriving from organ (visceral) disease or dysfunction.

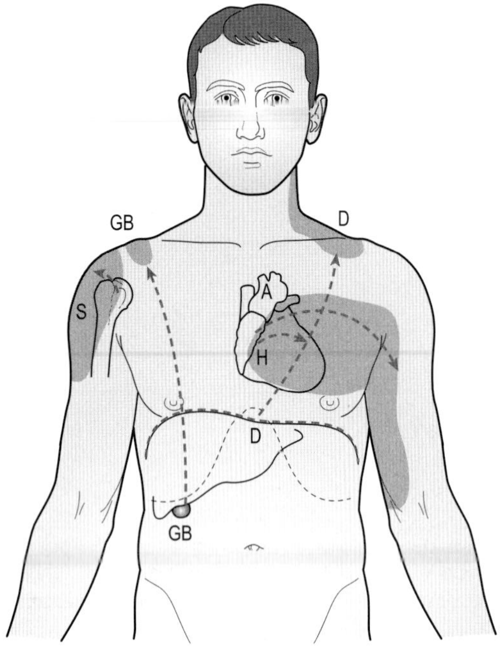

Figure 4.1   Visceral sources of shoulder pain. S, pain that originates in the shoulder; D, referred from diaphragm; H and A, axilla and pectoral pain referred from the heart; GB, pain referred from the gallbladder, which also extends posteriorly into the scapular region. (Reproduced with permission, from Chaitow & DeLany 2005, after Cailliet 1991.)

The importance of this information is that you might at first mistakenly think that pain in these areas is purely musculoskeletal.

It is important to rule out organ disease before treating pain problems that *might* be coming from other sources – but may also be the result of trigger point activity as described in earlier chapters.

This calls for careful case history taking and, if necessary, referral to a physician or other healthcare provider, to rule out stomach, gallbladder or other sources of the pain.

If you have a sense of unease about the cause(s) of a patient's symptoms you should play safe, for the sake of the patient and yourself, and make sure the patient is thoroughly checked before you start treatment.

PELVIC PAIN, INTERSTITIAL (UNEXPLAINED) CYSTITIS AND URINARY (STRESS) INCONTINENCE

Pelvic pain, and problems of urgency and incontinence, may at times be related to trigger points.

And of course there may be many other causes of these symptoms, including infection, gynecological disease, pregnancy, weight problems, etc.

As far back as the early 1950s there were reports that symptoms such as cystitis could be created by trigger points in the abdominal muscles (Kelsey 1951).

Travell & Simons (1982), the leading researchers into trigger points, reported that:

> Urinary frequency, urinary urgency and 'kidney' pain may be referred from trigger points in the skin of the lower abdominal muscles. Injection of an old appendectomy scar … has relieved frequency and urgency, and increased the bladder capacity significantly.

More recent research confirms this, and has shown that symptoms such as cystitis can often be relieved manually, as well as by injection (Oyama et al 2004, Weiss 2001) to deactivate trigger points.

IMPOSTER SYMPTOMS

Grieve (1994) has described 'imposter' symptoms:

> If we take patients off the street, we need more than ever to be awake to those conditions which may be other than musculoskeletal; this is not 'diagnosis', only an enlightened awareness of when manual or other physical therapy may be more than merely unsuitable and perhaps foolish. There is also the possibility of delaying more appropriate treatment.

Grieve suggests that we should be suspicious of symptoms that present as musculoskeletal if:

- the symptoms don't seem 'quite right', for example if there is a difference between the patient's story and the presenting symptoms
- the patient reports patterns of activity that aggravate or ease the symptoms which are unusual in your experience.

You should also be aware that symptoms that arise from sinister causes (cancer, for example) may mimic musculoskeletal symptoms, or may coexist with actual musculoskeletal problems.

If a treatment plan is not working out, if there is lack of progress, or if there are unusual responses to treatment, you should review the situation.

Examples

Numerous examples can be found of symptoms that mimic or cause back pain, or that relate to trigger point activity:

- Almost any abdominal disorder can refer pain to the back (peptic ulcer, colon cancer, abdominal arterial disease).

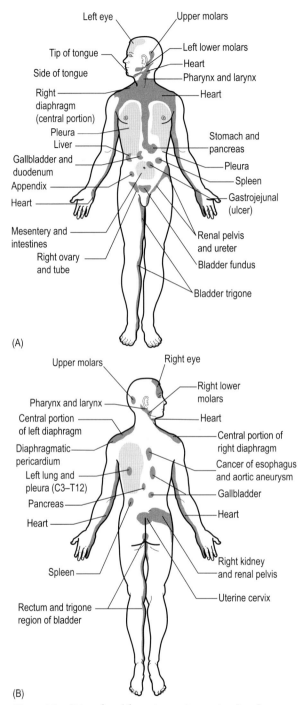

Labels, anterior view (A):
Left eye · Upper molars · Tip of tongue · Left lower molars · Side of tongue · Heart · Pharynx and larynx · Right diaphragm (central portion) · Heart · Pleura · Liver · Stomach and pancreas · Gallbladder and duodenum · Pleura · Appendix · Spleen · Heart · Gastrojejunal (ulcer) · Mesentery and intestines · Renal pelvis and ureter · Right ovary and tube · Bladder fundus · Bladder trigone

(A)

Labels, posterior view (B):
Upper molars · Right eye · Pharynx and larynx · Right lower molars · Central portion of left diaphragm · Heart · Diaphragmatic pericardium · Central portion of right diaphragm · Left lung and pleura (C3–T12) · Cancer of esophagus and aortic aneurysm · Pancreas · Gallbladder · Heart · Heart · Spleen · Right kidney and renal pelvis · Uterine cervix · Rectum and trigone region of bladder

(B)

Figure 4.2 Pain referred from viscera. A: anterior view. B: posterior view. (Reproduced with permission, from Chaitow & DeLany 2000, adapted from Rothstein et al 1991.)

- A hiatal hernia commonly produces bilateral thoracic and shoulder pain.
- Cauda equina syndrome (involving a cluster of fine nerves at the very end of the spinal cord) and/or other widespread neurological disorders, should be considered for the patient with low back pain who reports difficulty with urinating, and/or fecal incontinence (Waddell 1998). A 'saddle' shaped area of anesthesia may be reported around the anus, perineum or genitals, and there may be accompanying weakness in the legs, with obvious difficulties in walking. Immediate referral to a specialist is called for with any such symptoms.
- There should be suspicion of ankylosing spondylitis, or other chronic inflammatory conditions, if symptoms of progressive chronic low backache started before the age of 40 (usually in a male) and there is also: a family history; extreme stiffness in the morning; constant stiffness involving all movements of the spine in all directions; peripheral joint pain and restriction; associated colitis, iritis and/or skin problems such as psoriasis.
- Angina pain classically presents with chest, anterior cervical and (usually left) arm pain. Thoracic facet or disc conditions can mimic angina, as can active trigger point activity.
- Gallbladder problems commonly refer pain to the mid-thoracic area uni- or bilaterally. Suspicion should be aroused if eating makes the pain worse.
- Sacroiliac and right buttock pain may be produced by perforation of the ilium in regional ileitis (Crohn's disease).
- Pain similar to acute thoracolumbar dysfunction can be the result of stones in the ureter ('renal colic').
- Sudden severe low back pain (specially if the pain affects the testicles) may be associated with an aneurysm that is about to rupture (Grieve 1994).
- Trigger points are commonly found in quadratus lumborum in association with an irritated lumbar disc.
- Gluteal trigger points are often associated with hip joint pathology.

These examples of organ dysfunction or disease that mimics trigger point symptoms can also be reversed. There are often trigger point symptoms that seem very much like organ dysfunction. Because most massage therapists are not trained to make a diagnosis – and in many parts of the world (such as the USA), are expressly not allowed to do so – it is important to maintain an active, alert, suspicion about symptoms that don't 'seem quite right'.

SOME CHARACTERISTICS OF ABDOMINAL MUSCLE TRIGGER POINTS

Trigger points and abdominal pain

Sometimes abdominal pain that *feels* like organ dysfunction (stomach ache or cramp-like colon pain, for example) actually comes from trigger points in the abdominal muscles.

Some features of abdominal wall pain caused by trigger points are:

- Pain may be constant or fluctuating (comes and goes) and sometimes episodic (e.g. only during menstruation, or just before it).
- Pain intensity may be linked to postural positions (e.g. worse, or only when, lying, sitting or standing).
- Abdominal wall trigger point pain is not usually related to meals or bowel function.
- If a trigger point is responsible then there will be no findings of intra-abdominal causes for the symptoms.
- If abdominal tenderness remains unchanged, or actually increases, when the abdominal wall is tensed (if the patient raises his legs during palpation, for example), this suggests that the problem lies in the muscles and not the organ. This is a useful way of distinguishing between superficial (muscle) or deep (organ) causes of abdominal pain.
- Localized trigger points can usually be identified, often lying along the lateral margins of rectus abdominis or at the attachments of muscle or fascia.

BEST PRACTICE

And of course it is quite possible for someone to have organ dysfunction AND trigger point activity at the same time, with some pain/discomfort coming from one source and some from the other.

By suggesting that the patient has a thorough medical evaluation before you attempt to deactivate trigger points that may be adding to the symptoms, you will be protecting everyone's interests.

SCAR TISSUE AND TRIGGER POINTS

Trigger points may form in almost any body soft tissues; however, only those occurring in myofascial structures (muscle or fascia) are called 'myofascial trigger points'.

Trigger points are also found in skin, ligaments, joints, capsules and on the periosteum – the surface of bone where tendons attach.

And, as reported above, triggers often form in scar tissues (Simons et al 1999) from where they may produce and perpetuate pain for many years.

Scar tissue might also block normal lymphatic drainage (Chikly 1997), leading to a build-up of waste products in surrounding tissue that may encourage trigger point formation or recurrence.

Manual release of scar-related trigger points

Lewit & Olsanska (2004) report that they have been able to release numerous irritated, scar-related, trigger points, using gentle soft tissue methods (described in Chapter 7). They discuss over 50 cases, mainly female) aged between 16 and 85 years, with an average age of 50.

All the patients had severe chronic myofascial pain, involving a wide range of areas, including low back pain (14 patients), other back pain (4 patients), pain in the arm and shoulder (14 patients), headache (8 patients), neck pain (3 patients), pain in the thoracic region (3 patients), abdominal pain (2 patients). Three of the cases were treated for vertigo.

The trigger point-related scars, which were associated with the pain symptoms, were the result of either surgery (the majority), or injury.

What is important from this information is that wherever possible, when pain is a symptom, scars should be evaluated for trigger point activity (methods of assessment are described in Chapter 6).

If symptoms can be provoked during palpation assessment, treatment using soft tissue methods, as described in Chapter 7, is recommended. If these fail then a practitioner who uses injections or acupuncture should be considered for referral.

See also notes in Box 9.7, Chapter 9, on possible use of capsaicin cream in treating trigger points close to scar tissue.

TRIGGER POINTS AND JOINT RESTRICTION

Fortunately trigger points that occur in named specific muscles always refer to more or less the same target areas in everyone who has such triggers.

Scalene trigger points will always refer to the arm, gastrocnemius trigger points will always refer toward the ankle, and so on.

The key trigger points listed in the previous chapter (see Table 3.1) will always refer to the areas described, where satellite triggers develop.

Knowing this helps you to identify where pain or restriction may be coming from.

Trigger points in the muscles attaching to, or responsible for moving joints, can lead to loss of range of motion of those joints.

This means that the muscles that are associated with a particular joint's movement or stability, and that also house trigger points, are the ones in most need of assessment and treatment.

The muscles to which referral or radiating symptoms spread from trigger points in other muscles, can also restrict or cause pain in joints with which they are associated. For example, if a trigger point in the neck refers pain toward the scapula area, the local muscles in the referral zone (attaching to the scapula) will start to disturb normal movement of that important structure.

The maps later in this chapter (Figs 4.3 to 4.9) show the target areas influenced by particular trigger points in named muscles, so that choices can be made as to where to search for possible culprit triggers.

Any joint where there is a restriction of movement should be examined for trigger point involvement – and if the muscles that control the joint house triggers, or if pain is being radiated to, or referred into, any of the muscles that control the joint, the trigger point activity may be totally, or partially, responsible for the joint restriction.

Table 4.1 describes the likely muscles that would be housing trigger points related to particular restricted movements (Kuchera & McPartland 1997).

The body and region maps illustrated in this chapter should allow you to trace those muscles associated with pain and restriction in all areas, and most joints of the body.

Simons' observations

Simons and colleagues have outlined some common trigger points that are responsible for common musculoskeletal problems (Table 4.2) (Simons et al 1999).

MAPS

Much of the remainder of this chapter comprises maps showing areas affected by trigger points, along with lists of muscles that are commonly associated with those areas.

It is important to remember that although trigger points may be actively producing referred or radiating pain in the tissues that are highlighted in the body maps, there are numerous other causes of pain possible in these tissues. Particular attention should be paid to the possibility of organ (visceral) referral of pain, as well as 'imposter' symptoms.

It is safe to say that almost all chronic pain has, as part of its make-up, trigger point involvement – even if these are not the original cause of the pain (Wall & Melzack 1990).

Table 4.1 Muscles housing trigger points that may be related to restricted shoulder movements

Restricted shoulder motion	Muscle housing trigger point
Flexion	Subscapularis
	Infraspinatus
	Supraspinatus
Abduction	Triceps
	Teres major
	Levator scapulae
Internal rotation	Teres major
	Infraspinatus
External rotation	Subscapularis
	Pectoralis minor

Table 4.2 Common trigger point causes

Common diagnosis	Common trigger point causes
Tension-type headache	Sternocleidomastoid, upper trapezius, posterior cervical, temporalis
Frozen shoulder	Subscapularis, supraspinatus, pectoralis major and minor, deltoid muscles
Epicondylitis	Finger and hand extensors, supinator, and triceps brachii
Carpal tunnel syndrome	Scaleni, finger extensors
Atypical angina pectoris	Left pectoralis major, intercostals
Lower back pain	Quadratus lumborum, iliopsoas, thoracolumbar paraspinals, rectus abdominis, piriformis, gluteus maximus and medius

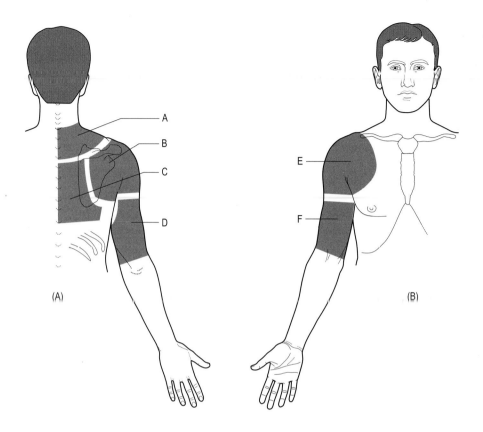

A. Upper-thoracic back pain
Scaleni
Levator scapulae
Supraspinatus
Trapezius
Multifidi
Rhomboidei
Splenius cervicis
Triceps brachii
Biceps brachii

B. Back-of-shoulder pain
Deltoid
Levator scapulae
Scaleni
Supraspinatus
Teres major
Teres minor
Subscapularis
Serratus posterior superior
Latissimus dorsi
Triceps brachii
Trapezius
Iliocostalis thoracis

C. Mid-thoracic back pain
Scaleni
Latissimus dorsi
Levator scapulae
Iliocostalis thoracis
Multifidi
Rhomboidei
Serratus posterior superior
Infraspinatus
Trapezius
Serratus anterior

D. Back-of-arm pain
Scaleni
Triceps brachii
Deltoid
Subscapularis
Supraspinatus
Teres major
Teres minor
Latissimus dorsi
Serratus posterior superior
Coracobrachialis
Scalenus minimus

E. Front-of-shoulder pain
Infraspinatus
Deltoid
Scaleni
Supraspinatus
Pectoralis major
Pectoralis minor
Biceps brachii
Coracobrachialis
Sternalis
Subclavius
Latissimus dorsi

F. Front-of-arm pain
Scaleni
Infraspinatus
Biceps brachii
Brachialis
Triceps brachii
Supraspinatus
Deltoid
Sternalis
Scalenus minimus
Subclavius

Figure 4.3 Designated areas in the shoulder and arm to which pain may be referred by myofascial trigger points. See listing of muscles that refer pain to each of these areas. (Reproduced with permission, from Chaitow & DeLany 2005, after Simons et al 1999.)

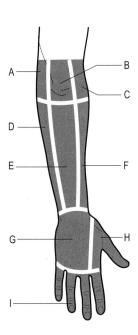

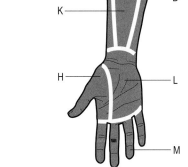

A. Medial epicondylar pain
Triceps brachii
Pectoralis major
Pectoralis minor
Serratus anterior
Serratus posterior superior

B. Olecranon pain
Triceps brachii
Serratus posterior superior

C. Lateral epicondylar pain
Supinator
Brachiordialis
Extensor carpi radialis longus
Triceps brachii
Supraspinatus
Fourth and fifth finger extensors
Anconeus

D. Ulnar forearm pain
Latissimus dorsi
Pectoralis major
Pectoralis minor
Serratus posterior superior

E. Dorsal forearm pain
Triceps brachii
Teres major
Extensor carpi radialis longus
  and brevis
Coracobrachialis
Scalenus minimus

F. Radial forearm pain
Infraspinatus
Scaleni
Brachiordialis
Supraspinatus
Subclavius

G. Dorsal wrist and hand pain
Extensor carpi radialis brevis
Extensor carpi radialis longus
Extensor digitorum
Extensor indicis
Extensor carpi ulnaris
Subscapularis
Coracobrachialis
Scalenus minimus
Latissimus dorsi
Serratus posterior superior
First dorsal interosseus

H. Base-of-thumb and radial hand pain
Supinator
Scaleni
Brachialis
Infraspinatus
Extensor carpi radialis longus
Brachiordialis
Opponens pollicis
Adductor pollicis
Subclavius
First dorsal interosseus
Flexor pollicis longus

I. Dorsal finger pain
Extensor digitorum
Interossei
Scaleni
Abductor digiti minimi
Pectoralis major
Pectoralis minor
Latissimus dorsi
Subclavius

J. Antecubital pain
Brachialis
Biceps brachii

K. Volar forearm pain
Palmaris longus
Pronator teres
Serratus anterior
Triceps brachii

L. Volar wrist and palmar pain
Flexor carpi radialis
Flexor carpi ulnaris
Opponens pollicis
Pectoralis major
Pectoralis minor
Latissimus dorsi
Palmaris longus
Pronator teres
Serratus anterior

M. Volar finger pain
Flexors digitorum superficialis
Flexor digitorum profundus
Interossei
Latissimus dorsi
Serratus anterior
Abductor digiti minimi
Subclavius

Figure 4.4   Designated areas in the forearm and hand region to which pain may be referred by myofascial trigger points. See listing of muscles that refer pain to each of these areas. (Reproduced with permission, from Chaitow & DeLany 2005, after Simons et al 1999.)

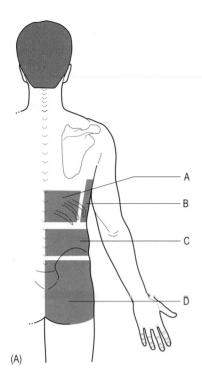

(A)

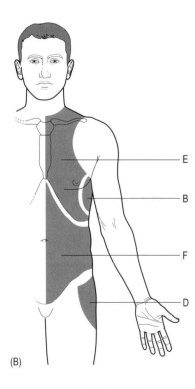

(B)

A. Low thoracic back pain
  Iliocostalis thoracis
  Multifidi
  Serratus posterior inferior
  Rectus abdominis
  Intercostals
  Latissimus dorsi
  Iliopsoas

B. Side-of-chest pain
  Serratus anterior
  Intercostals
  Latissimus dorsi
  Diaphragm

C. Lumbar pain
  Longissimus thoracis
  Iliocostalis lumborum
  Iliocostalis thoracis
  Multifidi
  Rectus abdominis
  Iliopsoas
  Gluteus medius

D. Sacral and gluteal pain
  Longissimus thoracis
  Iliocostalis lumborum
  Multifidi
  Quadratus lumborum
  Piriformis
  Gluteus medius
  Gluteus maximus
  Levator ani
  Obturator internus
  Gluteus minimus
  Sphincter ani
  Coccygeus
  Soleus

E. Front-of-chest pain
  Pectoralis major
  Pectoralis minor
  Scaleni
  Sternocleidomastoid (sternal)
  Sternalis
  Intercostals
  Iliocostalis cervicis
  Subclavius
  External abdominal oblique
  Diaphragm

F. Abdominal pain
  Rectus abdominis
  Abdominal obliques
  Transverse abdominis
  Iliocostalis thoracis
  Multifidi
  Pyramidalis
  Quadratus lumborum

Figure 4.5   Designated areas in the torso region to which pain may be referred by myofascial trigger points. See listing of muscles that refer pain to each of these areas. (Reproduced with permission, from Chaitow & DeLany 2005, after Simons et al 1999.)

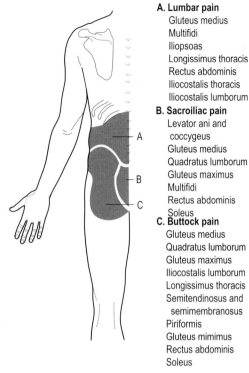

A. Lumbar pain
Gluteus medius
Multifidi
Iliopsoas
Longissimus thoracis
Rectus abdominis
Iliocostalis thoracis
Iliocostalis lumborum

B. Sacroiliac pain
Levator ani and
  coccygeus
Gluteus medius
Quadratus lumborum
Gluteus maximus
Multifidi
Rectus abdominis
Soleus

C. Buttock pain
Gluteus medius
Quadratus lumborum
Gluteus maximus
Iliocostalis lumborum
Longissimus thoracis
Semitendinosus and
  semimembranosus
Piriformis
Gluteus mimimus
Rectus abdominis
Soleus

Figure 4.6 Designated areas in the lumbar, sacroiliac, and buttock region to which pain may be referred by myofascial trigger points. See listing of muscles that refer pain to each of these areas. (Reproduced with permission, from Chaitow & DeLany 2005, after Travell & Simons 1992.)

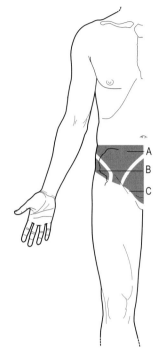

A. Abdominal pain
Rectus abdominis
Obliquus externus
  abdominis
Iliocostalis thoracis
Multifidi
Quadratus lumborum
Pyramidalis

B. Buttock pain
Gluteus medius
Quadratus lumborum
Gluteus maximus
Iliocostalis lumborum
Longissimus thoracis
Semitendinosus and
  semimembranosus
Piriformis
Gluteus minimus
Rectus abdominis
Soleus

C. Pelvic pain
Coccygeus
Levator ani
Obturator internus
Adductor magnus
Piriformis

Figure 4.7 Designated areas in the anterior abdominal and pelvic region to which pain may be referred by myofascial trigger points. See listing of muscles that refer pain to each of these areas. (Reproduced with permission, from Chaitow & DeLany 2005, after Travell & Simons 1992.)

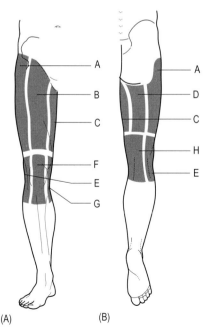

A. Lateral thigh and hip pain
Gluteus minimus
Vastus lateralis
Pirifomis
Quadratus lumborum
Tensor fasciae latae
Vastus intermedius
Gluteus maximus
Rectus femoris

B. Anterior thigh pain
Rectus femoris
Vastus medialis
Adductors longus and brevis

C. Medial thigh pain
Pectineus
Vastus medialis
Gracilis
Adductor magnus
Sartorius

D. Posterior thigh pain
Gluteus minimus
Semitendinosus and
  semimembranosus
Biceps femoris
Piriformis
Obturator internus

E. Lateral knee pain
Vastus lateralis

F. Anterior knee pain
Rectus femoris
Vastus medialis
Adductors longus and brevis

G. Anteromedial knee pain
Vastus medialis
Gracilis
Rectus femoris
Sartorius, lower TrP
Adductors longus and brevis

H. Posterior knee pain
Gastrocnemius
Biceps femoris
Popliteus
Semitendinosus and
  semimembranosus
Soleus
Plantaris

(A)   (B)

Figure 4.8 Designated areas in the anterior and posterior thigh region to which pain may be referred by myofascial trigger points. See listing of muscles that refer pain to each of these areas. (Reproduced with permission, from Chaitow & DeLany 2005, after Travell & Simons 1992.)

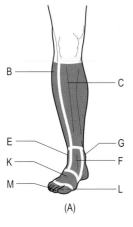

(A)

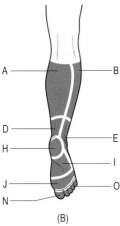

(B)

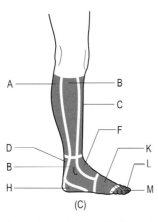

(C)

A. Posterior leg pain
Soleus
Gluteus minimus, posterior section
Gastrocnemius
Semitendinosus and semimembranosus
Flexor digitorum longus
Tibialis posterior
Plantaris

B. Lateral leg pain
Gastrocnemius
Gluteus minimus, anterior section
Peroneus longus and brevis
Vastus lateralis

C. Anterior leg pain
Tibialis anterior
Adductors longus and brevis

D. Posterior ankle pain
Soleus
Tibialis anterior

E. Lateral ankle pain
Peronei longus and brevis
Peroneus tertius

F. Anterior ankle pain
Tibialis anterior
Peroneus tertius
Extensor digitorum longus
Extensor hallucis longus

G. Medial ankle pain
Abductor hallucis
Flexor digitorum longus

H. Heel pain
Soleus
Quadratus plantae
Abductor hallucis
Tibialis posterior

I. Plantar midfoot pain
Gastrocnemius
Flexor digitorum longus
Adductor hallucis
Soleus
Interossei of foot
Abductor hallucis
Tibialis posterior

J. Metatarsal head pain
Flexor hallucis brevis
Flexor digitorum brevis
Adductor hallucis
Flexor hallucis longus
Interossei of foot
Abductor digiti minimi
Flexor digitorum longus
Tibialis posterior

K. Dorsal forefoot pain
Extensor digitorum brevis
and extensor hallucis brevis
Extensor digitorum longus
Extensor hallucis longus
Flexor hallucis brevis
Interossei of foot
Tibialis anterior

L. Dorsal great toe pain
Tibialis anterior
Extensor hallucis longus
Flexor hallucis brevis

M. Dorsal lesser toe pain
Interossei of foot
Extensor digitorum longus

N. Plantar great toe pain
Flexor hallucis longus
Flexor hallucis brevis
Tibialis posterior

O. Plantar lesser toe pain
Flexor digitorum longus
Tibialis posterior

Figure 4.9 Designated areas in the leg and foot to which pain may be referred by myofascial trigger points. See listing of muscles that refer pain to each of these areas. (Reproduced with permission, from Chaitow & DeLany 2005, after Travell & Simons 1992.)

NECK, HEAD AND FACE REFERRAL PATTERNS AND MAJOR TRIGGER POINT LOCATIONS

The maps illustrated below cover most of the body apart from the upper neck, head and face.

In the last section of this chapter some of the most important trigger points affecting those areas (face/head, etc.) are illustrated, together with their referral patterns.

These illustrations are all taken from *Clinical Applications of Neuromuscular Techniques Volume 1, Upper Body*, where detailed instructions are given for assessment and treatment of these (Chaitow & DeLany 2000).

Splenius capitis

There are two major trigger point sites in this muscle, capable of referring pain to the top and side of the head (upper point) as well as into the lateral aspects of the neck (lower point) (Fig. 4.10).

Suboccipital and semispinalis capitis

The trigger points in the suboccipital and semispinalis capitis muscles refer in a very similar pattern to the upper splenius – across the side of the head just above ear level to the forehead (Fig. 4.11).

See also Figure 6.17 for the referral zone of central upper trapezius trigger points.

Platysma

Referral from platysma trigger points is similar to part of the sternomastoid referral zone (see below) into the face (Fig. 4.12).

Sternocleidomastoid

There are numerous potential trigger point sites in sternocleidomastoid (SCM) (Fig. 4.13), requiring careful assessment (see Chapter 6), usually using a flat pincer grip (see Fig. 6.2).

Temporalis

A variety of trigger point sites in the enormously powerful temporalis muscle refer into different areas of the face, head and jaw (including the teeth) (Fig. 4.14).

Masseter

Masseter trigger points refer into the teeth, jaw, face and sinuses (Fig. 4.15).

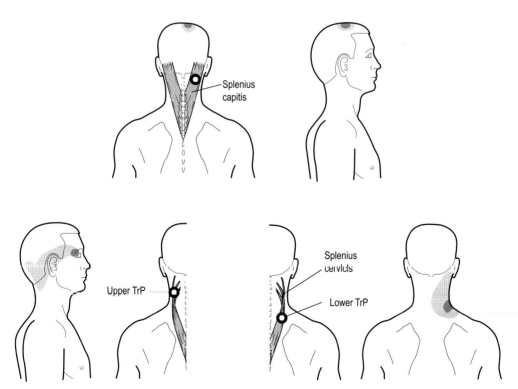

Figure 4.10 The combined patterns of splenii trigger point target zones of referral. (From Chaitow & DeLany 2000.)

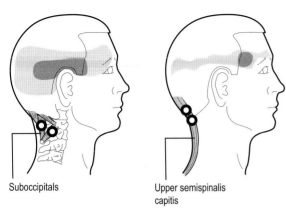

Suboccipitals

Upper semispinalis capitis

Figure 4.11   The referral patterns of the suboccipital muscles and the upper semispinalis capitis are similar. (From Chaitow & DeLany 2000.)

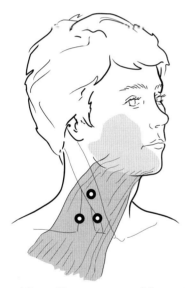

Figure 4.12   The prickling pain pattern of platysma is distinct from the pattern of the underlying SCM (see Fig. 4.13). (From Chaitow & DeLany 2000.)

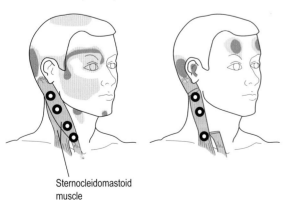

Sternocleidomastoid muscle

Figure 4.13   Composite referral patterns of SCM muscle. (From Chaitow & DeLany 2000.)

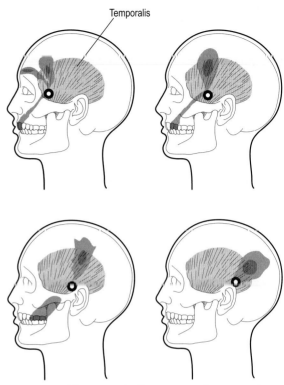

Temporalis

Figure 4.14   The temporalis fibers are vertically orientated anteriorly and horizontally oriented posteriorly, with varying diagonal fibers in between. (From Chaitow & DeLany 2000.)

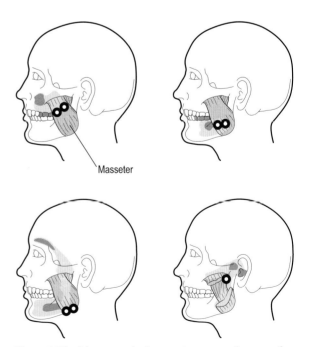

Masseter

Figure 4.15   Masseter and other masticatory muscles may refer directly into the teeth, creating pain or sensitivity. (From Chaitow & DeLany 2000.)

CLINICAL NOTE

Key points from Chapter 4

1. Many muscle and joint pains derive from organ dysfunction or disease. These should be ruled out before assuming that a particular pain is caused by trigger points.

2. It is always important to be suspicious of symptoms that don't quite make sense. Imposter symptoms should be considered, and a referral made to clarify the situation before treatment is started.

3. Even if the main source of pain is a diseased organ, some of the pain may be caused by trigger points, and as long as the main problem is being dealt with medically, it is quite in order to relieve the myofascial pain manually as long as all normal precautions are taken not to aggravate underlying problems.

4. Many pains arise from trigger points associated with scar tissue. All scars should be investigated (see Chapter 6) for possible links to pain.

5. Joint dysfunction may be connected to trigger point activity. Use maps to guide you to possible culprit muscles.

References

Cailliet R 1991 Shoulder pain. F A Davis, Philadelphia

Chaitow L, DeLany J 2000 Clinical applications of neuromuscular techniques. Vol 1, Upper body. Churchill Livingstone, Edinburgh

Chaitow L, DeLany J 2005 Clinical application of neuromuscular techniques. Practical case study exercises. Churchill Livingstone, Edinburgh

Chikly B 1997 Lymph drainage therapy study guide level II. Chikly and UI Publishing, Florida

Grieve G 1994 The masqueraders. In: Boyling J D, Palastanga N (eds) Grieve's modern manual therapy of the vertebral column, 2nd edn. Churchill Livingstone, Edinburgh

Kelsey M 1951 Diagnosis of upper abdominal pain. Texas State Journal of Medicine 47:82–86

Kuchera M, McPartland J 1997 Myofascial trigger points. In: Ward R (ed) Foundations of osteopathic medicine. Williams & Wilkins, Baltimore

Lewit K, Olsanska S 2004 Clinical importance of active scars: abnormal scars as a cause of myofascial pain. Journal of Manipulative and Physiological Therapeutics 27(6):399–402

Oyama I, Rejba A, Lukban J et al 2004 Modified Thiele massage as therapeutic intervention for female patients with interstitial cystitis and high-tone pelvic floor dysfunction. Urology 64(5):862–865

Rothstein J, Roy S H, Wolf S L 1999 Rehabilitation specialists handbook. F A Davis, Philadelphia

Simons J, Travell J, Simons L 1999 Myofascial pain and dysfunction: the trigger point manual. Vol 1, Upper body, 2nd edn. Williams & Wilkins, Baltimore

Travell J, Simons D 1983 Myofascial pain and dysfunction: the trigger point manual. Vol 1, Upper body, 1st edn. Williams & Wilkins, Baltimore, p 671

Travell J, Simons D 1992 Myofascial pain and dysfunction. Lower body. Williams & Wilkins, Baltimore

Waddell G 1998 The back pain revolution. Churchill Livingstone, Edinburgh

Wall P, Melzack R 1990 Textbook of pain, 2nd edn. Churchill Livingstone, Edinburgh

Weiss J 2001 Pelvic floor myofascial trigger points: manual therapy for interstitial cystitis and the urgency-frequency syndrome. Journal of Urology 166:2226–2231

CHAPTER FIVE

'Measuring the pain'

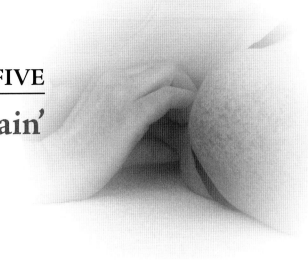

How much pain is the patient experiencing? Before looking at what we can see and touch – the observable and palpable characteristics of trigger points, in Chapter 6 – it is important to discuss how to assess and record the patient's pain experience.

Pain thresholds differ from person to person, and in the same person, depending on, among other things, how worried the person is about the pain.

A stomach-ache after overeating will be less worrisome than a stomach-ache that has no obvious cause, especially if someone you know has recently been diagnosed with abdominal cancer!

While one person may report a muscle or joint as being painful, someone else might report the very same degree of pain as discomfort.

There are cultural, as well as physiological, ethnic and gender reasons for this (Melzack & Katz 1999).

It may be surprising to learn that women, on average, have a far lower pain threshold than men.

Wolfe and colleagues (1995) showed that although approximately 60% of women can tolerate 4 kilos (8 lb) of pressure before reporting pain, approximately 90% of men can tolerate this amount of pressure without feeling what they would describe as pain.

Less than 5% of women can tolerate 12 kilos (25 lb) of pressure, while nearly 50% of men can do so.

This gender difference is well worth remembering when testing pain levels.

WHAT WE NEED TO KNOW

It is important to have ways of easily recording the person's present sense of pain, so that there is a record that can be compared with what is reported later.

We need to know:

- Where the pain is.
- What it feels like (words such as ache, sharp, burning, etc.).
- What other symptoms (inflammation, for example, or a fever) accompany the pain.
- Whether the symptoms are constant or fluctuating.
- What aggravates the pain and what makes it easier.
- The times of day when pain is most obvious. (In bed at night? When moving about? After moving about and sitting?)
- What activities are prevented by the pain ('I cannot (or it is difficult to) walk, sit down, carry anything, etc.').

There are a variety of 'tools' that can help to record pain symptoms, ranging from questionnaires to simple paper-based measuring scales, as well as instruments such as a pressure gauge, an algometer. There are various types of algometer. Some are simple, spring-loaded, hand-held devices, while others use digital technology. See later in this chapter for more on this useful instrument.

RATING SCALES

The simplest measuring device, the *verbal rating scale* (VRS), records on paper or a computer, what a patient reports – whether there is 'no pain', 'mild pain', 'moderate pain', 'severe pain' or 'agonizing pain' (Fig. 5.1A) (Jensen & Karoly 1991).

A *numerical rating scale* (NRS) uses a series of numbers (zero to 100, or zero to 10, for example), with no pain at all attached to the zero end, and 'the worst pain possible' attached to the highest number on the scale (Fig. 5.1B). The patient is asked to apply a

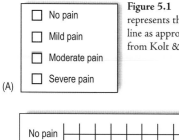

(A)

Figure 5.1   A: A verbal rating scale. The patient is instructed to mark the verbal description that best represents their pain. B: A numerical rating scale. The patient is instructed to mark the numbered vertical line as appropriate. C: A horizontal visual analogue scale for pain intensity. (Reproduced with permission, from Kolt & Andersen 2004.)

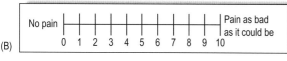

(B)

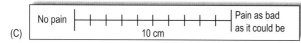

(C)

numerical value to the pain. This is noted down and recorded along with the date. Using an NRS is a common and quite accurate method for measuring the intensity of pain, but does not take account of factors other than intensity, such as the 'meaning' the patient gives to the pain (Melzack & Katz 1999).

The *visual analogue scale* (VAS) is a widely used method. This consists of a line drawn on paper that measures 10 centimeters, with marks at each end, and at each centimeter (Fig. 5.1C). Again the zero end of the line is marked as representing no pain at all, and the other end as representing the worst pain possible. The patient simply marks the line at the level of their pain. The VAS can be used to measure progress by comparing the pain scores over time. The VAS has been found to be accurate when used for anyone over the age of 5.

QUESTIONNAIRES

A variety of questionnaires exist such as the McGill Pain Questionnaire (Fig. 5.2A) and the Short-form McGill Pain Questionnaire (Fig. 5.2B). The shorter version offers a number of words that describe pain (such as throbbing, shooting, stabbing, heavy, sickening, fearful).

Use of such questionnaires requires some training so that accurate interpretation can be made of the patient's answers. Therefore, apart from acknowledging that they can be very useful, the McGill (and other) questionnaires will not be discussed in this book.

There are a number of ways of getting further information, the simplest being to conduct a web search using 'McGill questionnaire' as the key words.

PAIN DRAWINGS

It is useful to have the patient color the areas of their pain on a simple outline of the human body (a red pencil makes this more graphic) (Fig. 5.3A).

The patient can also be asked to write single word descriptions of the pain in different areas – throbbing, aching, etc., or to use a code in which (for example) xx = burning pain, !! = stabbing pain, 00 = aching, and so on.

This provides a record of both the location, and the nature, of the person's pain, and can usefully be repeated at future visits.

The shaded or colored areas can be very useful when searching for trigger points, in combination with the body maps provided in Chapter 4.

A single sheet of paper can easily contain a VAS, a shortened McGill Questionnaire, as well as a series of simple questions such as those illustrated in Figure 5.3B.

THE ALGOMETER

The art of palpation, and of applying pressure to treat tissues, requires sensitivity.

We need to be aware when tissue tension/resistance is being 'met', as we palpate, and when tension is being overcome.

When we palpate or apply digital pressure to a tender point, and ask 'Does it hurt?', 'Does it refer?', etc., it is important to have an idea of how much pressure is being applied.

The term 'pain threshold' is used to describe the least amount of pressure needed to produce a report of pain, and/or referred symptoms, when a trigger point is being compressed (Hong et al 1996).

■ McGill Pain Questionnaire ■

Patient's name _____ Date _____ Time _____ am/pm

PRI: S _____ A _____ E _____ M _____ PRI(T) _____ PPI _____
  (1–10)   (11–15)   (16)   (17–20)   (1–20)

1 FLICKERING   ___
  QUIVERING   ___
  PULSING   ___
  THROBBING   ___
  BEATING   ___
  POUNDING   ___
2 JUMPING   ___
  FLASHING   ___
  SHOOTING   ___
3 PRICKING   ___
  BORING   ___
  DRILLING   ___
  STABBING   ___
  LANCINATING   ___
4 SHARP   ___
  CUTTING   ___
  LACERATING   ___
5 PINCHING   ___
  PRESSING   ___
  GNAWING   ___
  CRAMPING   ___
  CRUSHING   ___
6 TUGGING   ___
  PULLING   ___
  WRENCHING   ___
7 HOT   ___
  BURNING   ___
  SCALDING   ___
  SEARING   ___
8 TINGLING   ___
  ITCHY   ___
  SMARTING   ___
  STINGING   ___
9 DULL   ___
  SORE   ___
  HURTING   ___
  ACHING   ___
  HEAVY   ___
10 TENDER   ___
  TAUT   ___
  RASPING   ___
  SPLITTING   ___
	11 TIRING ___
	  EXHAUSTING ___
	12 SICKENING ___
	  SUFFOCATING ___
	13 FEARFUL ___
	  FRIGHTFUL ___
	  TERRIFYING ___
	14 PUNISHING ___
	  GRUELLING ___
	  CRUEL ___
	  VICIOUS ___
	  KILLING ___
	15 WRETCHED ___
	  BLINDING ___
	16 ANNOYING ___
	  TROUBLESOME ___
	  MISERABLE ___
	  INTENSE ___
	  UNBEARABLE ___
	17 SPREADING ___
	  RADIATING ___
	  PENETRATING ___
	  PIERCING ___
	18 TIGHT ___
	  NUMB ___
	  DRAWING ___
	  SQUEEZING ___
	  TEARING ___
	19 COOL ___
	  COLD ___
	  FREEZING ___
	20 NAGGING ___
	  NAUSEATING ___
	  AGONIZING ___
	  DREADFUL ___
	  TORTURING ___
	PPI
	0 NO PAIN ___
	1 MILD ___
	2 DISCOMFORTING ___
	3 DISTRESSING ___
	4 HORRIBLE ___
	5 EXCRUCIATING ___

BRIEF	RHYTHMIC	CONTINUOUS
MOMENTARY	PERIODIC	STEADY
TRANSIENT	INTERMITTENT	CONSTANT

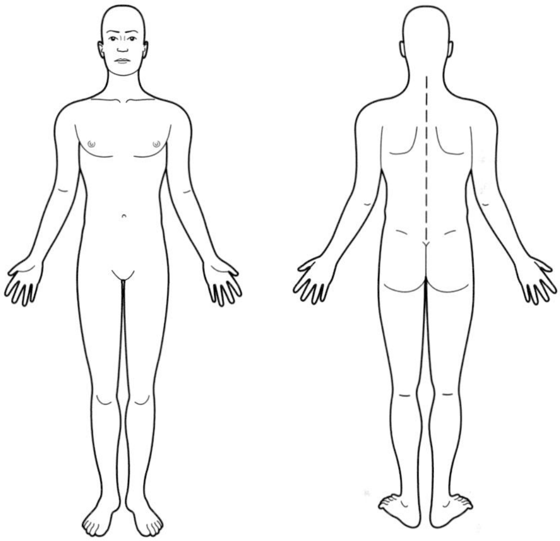

E = EXTERNAL

I = INTERNAL

COMMENTS:

(A)

Figure 5.2A McGill Pain Questionnaire. The descriptors fall into four major groups: sensory, 1–10; affective, 11–15; evaluative, 16; and miscellaneous, 17–20. The rank value for each descriptor is based on its position in the word set. The sum of the rank values is the pain rating index (PRI). The present pain intensity (PPI) is based on a scale of 0–5. (Reproduced with permission, from Melzack 1975.)

	NONE	MILD	MODERATE	SEVERE
	Short-form McGill Pain Questionnaire			
	Ronald Melzack			

Patient's name _____ Date _____

	NONE	MILD	MODERATE	SEVERE
THROBBING	0) _____	1) _____	2) _____	3) _____
SHOOTING	0) _____	1) _____	2) _____	3) _____
STABBING	0) _____	1) _____	2) _____	3) _____
SHARP	0) _____	1) _____	2) _____	3) _____
CRAMPING	0) _____	1) _____	2) _____	3) _____
GNAWING	0) _____	1) _____	2) _____	3) _____
HOT-BURNING	0) _____	1) _____	2) _____	3) _____
ACHING	0) _____	1) _____	2) _____	3) _____
HEAVY	0) _____	1) _____	2) _____	3) _____
TENDER	0) _____	1) _____	2) _____	3) _____
SPLITTING	0) _____	1) _____	2) _____	3) _____
TIRING-EXHAUSTING	0) _____	1) _____	2) _____	3) _____
SICKENING	0) _____	1) _____	2) _____	3) _____
FEARFUL	0) _____	1) _____	2) _____	3) _____
PUNISHING-CRUEL	0) _____	1) _____	2) _____	3) _____

No pain |————————————————————————————————| Worst possible pain

PPI
0 NO PAIN _____
1 MILD _____
2 DISCOMFORTING _____
3 DISTRESSING _____
4 HORRIBLE _____
5 EXCRUCIATING _____

(B)

Figure 5.2B   The Short-form McGill Pain Questionnaire. Descriptors 1–11 represent the sensory dimension of pain experience and 12–15 represent the affective dimension. Each descriptor is ranked on an intensity scale of 0 = none, 1 = mild, 2 = moderate, 3 = severe. The present pain intensity (PPI) of the standard long-form McGill Pain Questionnaire and the visual analogue scale are also included to provide overall pain intensity scores. (Reproduced with permission, from Melzack 1987.)

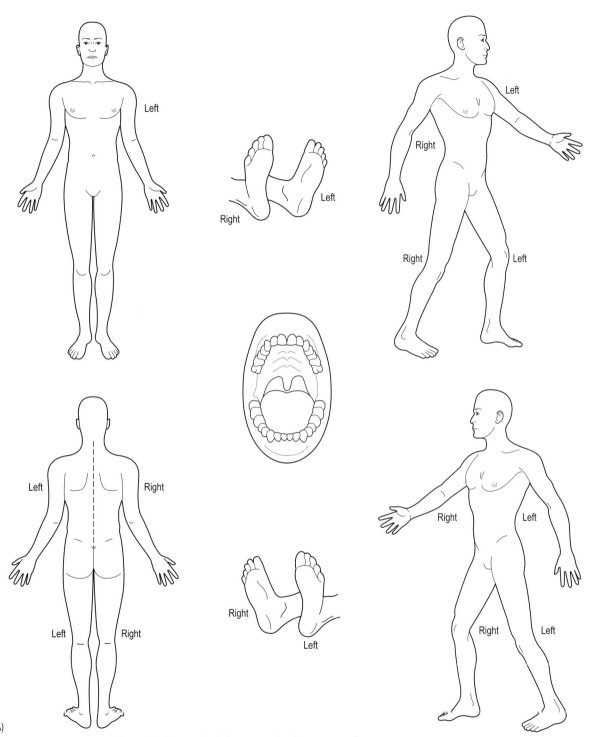

Figure 5.3A   Outlines of human body onto which the patient sketches patterns of pain.

NAME _____   DATE _____

Please tick any of the words that describes your pain
under the column that describes it's intensity.

PLEASE DRAW YOUR PAIN

	None	Mild	Moderate	Severe
Throbbing				
Shooting				
Stabbing				
Cramping				
Gnawing				
Hot-Burning				
Aching				
Heavy				
Tender				
Splitting				
Tiring-Exhausting				
Sickening				
Fearful				
Punishing-Cruel				

xxx	Burning	= =	Numbness
!!	Stabbing	**	Cramping
oo	Arching	?	Other

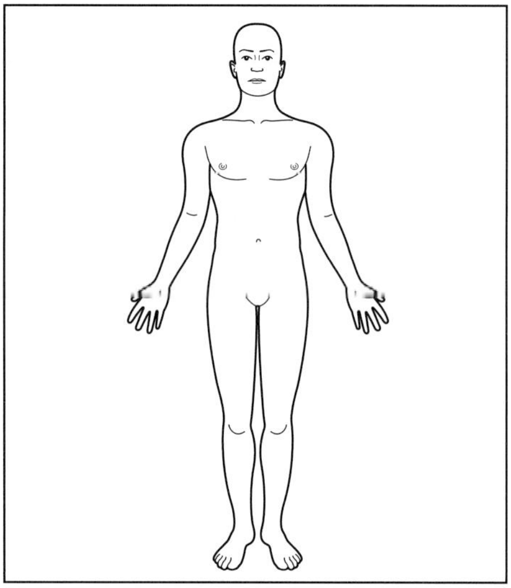

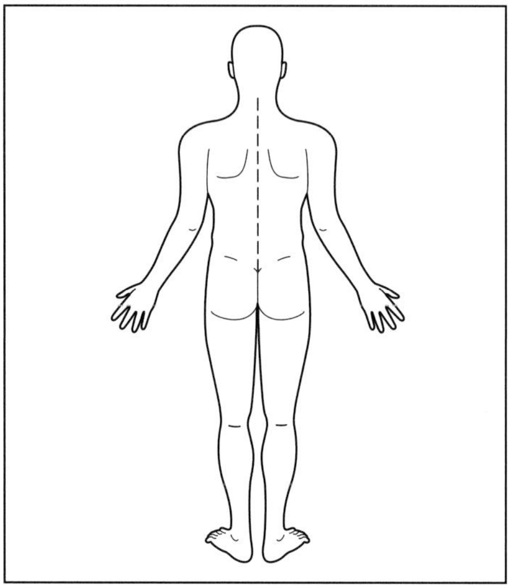

Your Pain is:

On Most Days ..... No Pain   Mild
                        Discomforting   Distressing
                        Horrible   Excruciating

At It's Worst .... No Pain   Mild
                        Discomforting   Distressing
                        Horrible   Excruciating

At It's Best .... No Pain   Mild
                        Discomforting   Distressing
                        Horrible   Excruciating

TODAY   No Pain   Mild
                        Discomforting   Distressing
                        Horrible   Excruciating

How many hours of the day are you in pain?   ....

How many days per week are you in pain?   ....

How many weeks per year are you in pain?   ....

What Drugs Have You Taken Today?   ....

....

Your Pain Today - Tick along scale below

No Pain [_____ **] Worst Possible Pain**

(B)

Figure 5.3B   Pain chart for gathering descriptive terms from the patient, and for sketching pain patterns.

It is obviously useful to know how much pressure is required to produce pain, and/or referred symptoms, and whether the amount of pressure being used has changed after treatment, or whether the pain threshold is different the next time the patient comes for treatment.

It would not be very helpful to hear: 'Yes it still hurts' only because we are pressing much harder.

Ideally, when testing for trigger point activity, we should be able to apply a moderate amount of force, just enough to cause no more than a sense of pressure in normal tissues, and to be always able to apply the same amount of effort whenever we test.

We should be able to apply enough pressure to produce the trigger point referral pain, and know that the same pressure, after treatment, no longer causes pain referral (Fryer & Hodgson 2005).

How can a person learn to apply a particular amount of pressure, and no more?

It has been shown that, using a simple technology (such as bathroom scales), physical therapy students can be taught to accurately produce specific degrees of pressure on request.

Students were tested applying pressure to lumbar muscles. After training, using bathroom scales, the students were able to apply precise amounts of pressure on request (Keating et al 1993).

Without a measuring device, such as an algometer, there would be no accurate way of achieving a standardized degree of pressure.

A basic algometer is a hand-held, spring-loaded, rubber-tipped, pressure-measuring device, which offers a means of achieving standardized pressure application. Using an algometer, sufficient pressure to produce pain is applied at preselected points, at a precise 90° angle to the skin. The measurement is taken when pain is reported.

An electronic version of this type of algometer allows recording of pressures applied. However, these forms of algometer are used independently of actual treatment, to obtain feedback from the patient, to register the pressure being used when pain levels reach tolerance, for example (Fig. 5.4A and B).

A variety of other algometer designs exist, including a sophisticated version that is attached to the thumb or finger, with a lead running to an electronic sensor that is itself connected to a computer. This gives very precise readouts of the amount of pressure being applied by the finger or thumb during treatment (Fig. 5.4C and D) (Fryer & Hodgson 2005).

Baldry (1993) suggests that algometers should be used to measure the degree of pressure required to produce symptoms, 'before and after deactivation of a trigger point, because when treatment is successful, the pressure threshold over the trigger point increases'.

If an algometer is not available, and in order to encourage only appropriate amounts of pressure being applied, it may be useful to practice simple palpation exercises.

TISSUE 'LEVELS'

Pick (1999) has useful suggestions regarding the levels of tissue that you should try to reach by application of pressure, in assessment and treatment.

He describes the different levels of tissues you should be aiming for:

Surface level: This is the first contact, molding to the contours of the structure, no actual pressure. This is just touching, without any pressure at all and is used to start treatment via the skin – as described in detail in Chapter 6.

Working level: Pick (1999) describes the working level as: 'the level at which most manipulative procedures begin. Within this level the practitioner can feel pliable counter-resistance to the applied force. The contact feels non-invasive … and is usually well within the comfort zone of the subjects. Here the practitioner will find maximum control over the intracranial structures.'

Rejection levels: Pick suggests these levels are reached when tissue resistance is overcome, and discomfort/pain is reported. Rejection will occur at different degrees of pressure, in different areas, and in different circumstances.

So how much pressure should be used?

1. When working with the skin: surface level.
2. When palpating for trigger points: working level.
3. When testing for pain responses, and when treating trigger points: rejection level.

When you are at the rejection level there is a feeling of the tissues pushing you away, you have to overcome the resistance to achieve a sustained compression, as described in Chapter 7.

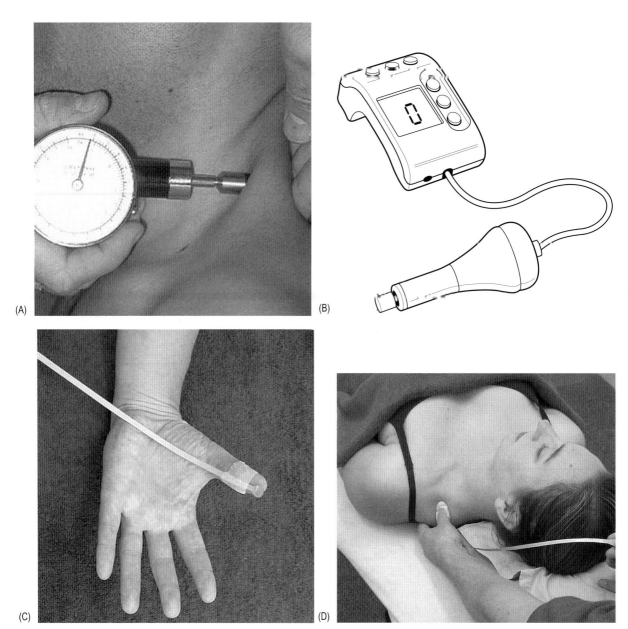

(A)

(B)

(C)

(D)

Figure 5.4 A: Mechanical pressure algometer being used to measure applied pressure. B: A version of an electronic algometer. C: Electronic algometer pressure pad attached to thumb (and to computer). D: Electronic algometer being used to evaluate pressure being applied to upper trapezius trigger point.

CLINICAL NOTE

Key points from Chapter 5

1. It is useful to have a record of the level of a patient's pain from the first visit, so that comparisons can be made over time.

2. There are a variety of ways of achieving a record, ranging from simple questions and answers to use of various scales and questionnaires.

3. The algometer (pressure gauge) is a tool that provides information as to how much pressure is needed to produce pain.

4. This information can and should be recorded so that progress (or no progress) can be measured accurately.

References

Baldry P 1993 Acupuncture, trigger points and musculoskeletal pain. Churchill Livingstone, Edinburgh

Fryer G, Hodgson L 2005 The effect of manual pressure release on myofascial trigger points in the upper trapezius muscle. Journal of Bodywork and Movement Therapies 9(4): in press

Hong C-Z, Chen Y-N, Twehouse D, Hong D 1996 Pressure threshold for referred pain by compression on trigger point and adjacent area. Journal of Musculoskeletal Pain 4(3):61–79

Jensen M, Karoly P 1991 Control beliefs, coping efforts and adjustments to chronic pain. Journal of Consulting and Clinical Psychology 59:431–438

Keating J, Matyas T A, Bach T M 1993 The effect of training on physical therapists' ability to apply specified forces of palpation. Physical Therapy 73(1):45–53

Kolt G, Andersen M 2004 Psychology in the physical and manual therapies. Churchill Livingstone, Edinburgh, p 151

Melzack R 1975 The McGill Pain Questionnaire: major properties and scoring methods. Pain 1:227–299

Melzack R 1987 The Short-form McGill Pain Questionnaire. Pain 30:191–197

Melzack R, Katz J 1999 Pain measurement in persons with pain. In: Wall P, Melzack R (eds) Textbook of pain, 4th edn. Churchill Livingstone, Edinburgh, p 409–420

Pick M 1999 Cranial sutures: analysis, morphology and manipulative strategies. Eastland Press, Seattle, p xx–xxi

Wolfe F, Ross K, Anderson J et al 1995 Aspects of fibromyalgia in the general population. Journal of Rheumatology 22:151–156

CHAPTER SIX

Finding trigger points by palpation

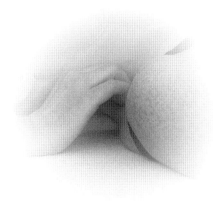

It is quite likely – almost inevitable – that during a regular massage treatment you will locate areas that are painful, and that also radiate or refer pain when pressed.

If this happens you will have discovered a trigger point, and because you know that active points are responsible for pain that the patient recognizes, as part of her symptoms, you will be able to tell the difference between active and latent points.

Because you will also know that central points lie in the bellies of muscles, while attachment points are close to attachments, you will be able to tell these apart.

But what if you do not 'trip over' trigger points during your massage treatment?

There are times when you may need to go looking for them.

There are likely to be times when you will suspect that a trigger point is responsible for a patient's pain symptoms. This is most likely when the patient complains of pain that keeps coming back, but for which there is no obvious cause.

And sometimes symptoms that are not painful might result from trigger points.

For example, digestive conditions might be the result of trigger points in one of the abdominal muscles, or increased nasal secretions could be the result of trigger points in muscles (such as sternomastoid) that refer into the sinus and nasal areas (Simons et al 1999). See later in this chapter for more on this, and also Figure 6.17B.

But how are you to locate the culprit trigger points? Where should you start searching?

QUESTIONS TO ASK

Before anything else a number of basic questions regarding the patient's pain need to be asked:

- Where is the pain? It is important to have the patient physically point to where the pain is experienced. All too often a comment such as it's 'in my hip (or kidney area)' means one thing to the patient, and quite another to you.
- Alternatively, have the patient draw the area of pain on a body outline as described in Chapter 5. Questions to ask include:
- Have you experienced these symptoms (this pain) before, or is this the first time you have experienced this?
- Describe the pain … what does it feel like? (Does it ache? Is it sharp?, etc.)
- If you have had this pain before, how long did it take to get better? (and was treatment needed? – and did it help? – and what sort of treatment was it?)
- How did the pain start?
- Does the pain spread, or is it localized?
- How long has the pain been there?
- Is it there all the time?
- If not when is the pain present/worst (at night, after activity, etc.)?
- What seems to aggravate it?
- 'What seems to ease it?'
- Does the pain prevent you from doing anything you would normally do?

The answers to these questions should be recorded in the notes, so that a month or six weeks down the line you can compare them with answers given then.

Changes in the answers offer evidence of change in the condition (as will changes in pain scores, etc., as outlined in Chapter 5).

STAR PALPATION

In osteopathic medicine the acronym STAR is used as a reminder of the characteristics of somatic dysfunction, such as myofascial trigger points.

STAR stands for:

- **S**ensitivity (or 'Tenderness') – this is the one feature that is almost always present when there is soft tissue dysfunction.
- **T**issue texture change – the tissues usually 'feel' different (for example they may be tense, fibrous, swollen, hot, cold or have other 'differences' from normal).
- **A**symmetry – there will commonly be an imbalance on one side, compared with the other, but this is not always the case.
- **R**ange of motion reduced – muscles will probably not be able to reach their normal resting length, or joints may have a restricted range.

The acronym is modified in some texts to TART (**T**enderness – **A**symmetry – **R**ange of movement modified – **T**issue texture change).

If two or three of these features are present this is enough to confirm that there is a problem, a dysfunction. It does not, however, explain why the problem exists, but is a start in the process toward understanding the patient's symptoms.

Research by Fryer et al (2004) has confirmed that this traditional osteopathic palpation method is valid. When tissues in the thoracic paraspinal muscles were found to be 'abnormal' (tense, dense, indurated), the same tissues (using an algometer) were also found to have a lowered pain threshold.

Less pressure was needed to create pain.

While the 'tenderness', altered texture and range of motion characteristics, as listed in the STAR (or TART) acronym, are *always* true for trigger points, additional trigger point changes have been listed by Simons and colleagues (1999):

- The soft tissues housing the trigger point will demonstrate a painful limit to stretch range of motion – whether the stretching is active, or passive (i.e. the patient is stretching the muscle, or you are stretching the muscle).

- In such muscles there is usually pain or discomfort when the muscle is contracted against resistance, with no movement taking place (i.e. an isometric contraction).
- The amount of force the muscle can generate is reduced when it contains active (or latent) trigger points – it is weaker than a normal muscle.
- A palpable taut band with an exquisitely tender nodule exists, and this should be found by palpation, unless the trigger lies in very deep muscle and is not accessible.
- Pressure on the tender spot produces pain familiar to the patient, and often a pain response ('jump sign').

SITES

Medical acupuncture expert Peter Baldry (1993) confirms what has already been described in previous chapters, that the commonest sites for trigger points are close to:

- muscular origins and insertions
- free borders of muscle
- muscle belly
- motor endpoint
- body tissues other than muscle, including skin, fascia, ligament, joint capsule, tendon and periosteum (and therefore 'attachment' areas), and also in scar tissue.

AN EXAMPLE

The patient should be asked to quantify the pain, as described in Chapter 5, using one or several of the methods mentioned there (scale of 0 to 10, for example, on a visual analogue scale).

Somewhere in the question and answer process you may start to suspect that trigger point activity may be involved.

Or you may have suspected this because of the patient's history and symptoms.

But how are you to know where to look?

The best and most accurate way is to work backwards from the area of reported pain (or other symptoms).

For example, consider a patient who reports an aching pain on the right side of the face, forehead, and around the ear (look at the 'maps' in Chapter 4).

- There may be no obvious problems in those areas, and no history pointing to an obvious reason for the pain.

- There may be no dental problems, no ear infection, no history of recent injuries, or of trauma in the past, that might help to explain this pain.
- The patient might have told you that the pain came on gradually over the past month or so, and seems to be worse during periods of stress.
- You may therefore be justified in thinking that this problem sounds as though it might involve trigger point activity.
- And because you know where the pain is located, and because trigger point patterns are consistent (the same trigger in different people refers – fairly closely – to the same target area) you can quickly find out where the likely trigger points feeding into that area will be, by looking at the 'maps' in Chapter 4.
- The most likely muscles are upper trapezius and/or sternomastoid, on the same side of the body as the pain. See Figure 6.17A, later in this chapter, for the referral pattern of a typical upper trapezius trigger point (and compare this with the acupuncture meridian pathway, as shown in Fig. 9.1 in Chapter 9).
- Your task will then be fairly simple – to locate a central, active trigger point in one of those muscles.
- When you locate the trigger (see Box 6.6), and press it, the pain that the patient is reporting should be reproduced.
- You need to ask: 'Does this hurt?'
- If the answer is 'yes', after a few more seconds of pressure, you would ask: 'Does the pain spread, or hurt you anywhere else, other than where I am pressing?'
- Again if the answer is something such as: 'Yes – that's making the side of my head ache just where it does when the pain comes on at work/home/ when driving', you will have confirmed that the trigger point was responsible for the 'familiar pain', you will have identified the source of the pain.

You may not yet have discovered *why* the particular muscle has been stressed enough to allow the trigger point to develop and become active, but you do at least know where the pain is coming from.

Among the other questions you might ask in order to discover background causes are:

- Have there been any new activities, new hobbies or changes in posture at work?
- Have you been spending more time typing, painting, lifting, gardening, reading, writing – or anything else that might place strain on these neck and shoulder muscles?
- Have you recently been under more stress than usual – and if so what kind?

- Have you recently had air-conditioning installed, or been in a draught?
- Have you recently taken a long-haul economy flight?
- … and/or carried luggage?

You should also evaluate posture, work and leisure activities, and breathing patterns, as discussed in earlier chapters.

There are *always* contributing and maintaining features that you may be able to identify and hopefully offer advice about, so that once the active trigger has been deactivated it does not simply come back again, because the causes have not been removed.

How do you go about locating the 'culprit' trigger point now that you know which muscles to search?

To explain this process it is necessary to restate the most important visible and palpable characteristics of

Cautions and contraindications

1. Before starting to palpate for trigger points you should have a reasonable idea of the nature and location (and ideally the causes) of your patient's symptoms.
2. And you should also have ruled out the possibility of potentially dangerous causes.
3. See, in particular, Chapter 4 for notes on 'imposter' symptoms.

It is also necessary to remember some basic contraindications to the use of manual pressure (or needles) to either identify, or to deactivate, trigger points:

- Be very cautious about deep pressure to identify or treat (deactivate) trigger points when pain is related to malignancy. Gentle approaches, such as lymphatic drainage, might be more appropriate in such situations. See later in this chapter for a reminder of how much pressure it is safe to use for assessment and for treatment.
- Avoid doing anything that involves deep pressure or stretching in the region of inflamed tissues.
- The same caution applies to areas where there are open wounds, or where there has been recent trauma (bruising, internal bleeding, torn tissues, fracture, etc.).
- Avoid deep tissue work (pressure, friction, stretching, etc.) anywhere near varicose veins, or if the patient has a history of atherosclerosis or aneurysm, or if the patient is taking blood-thinning (anticoagulant) medication for cardiovascular disease.

Cautions and contraindications – cont'd

- Be very cautious using stretching or deep pressure on patients with a diagnosis of osteoporosis, as bones may be so fragile that there would be risk of damage.
- Avoid deep tissue work of any sort in patients with a diagnosis of fibromyalgia, as the condition has as one of its symptoms very poor tissue repair potential (probably due to low levels of growth hormone). Deep work (or strong stretching) in such tissues creates microtrauma that may not easily be repaired.
- Avoid stretching, apart from very lightly, when the patient shows signs of hypermobility ('lax-joints'), as it is easy to create instability in already over-mobile structures.

trigger points, but before doing so it is essential to note some even more important cautions.

STARTING THE SEARCH

If you have decided which muscle(s) need to be searched for trigger points (based on the pain pattern and the maps) you might first consider just looking for altered skin status (see below for common signs) before starting to palpate.

Careful observation and palpation usually allows discovery of active trigger points in a fairly short space of time, 5 to 10 minutes at most.

This should allow ample time to start the process of deactivating the key points – as described in Chapter 7 – a process that takes approximately 4 to 7 minutes per trigger point, when working manually.

Needling a trigger point is faster, but is not necessarily more efficient (de las Peñas et al 2005).

Remember to look back at the list of 'key' points (Table 3.1, Chapter 3) that may be maintaining satellite points in an active state. This can save a lot of time and effort.

What does the tissue above a trigger point look like?

There are sometimes observable changes on the skin above trigger points:

1. Orange peel skin (also called 'goose-skin') may be seen above a trigger point, or in the target zone.
2. There may be localized edema (tissue swelling) that is visible locally in the area of the trigger point.

3. Cellulite may be apparent in the tissues above a trigger point.
4. There is almost always increased sympathetic activity in the tissues surrounding and above a trigger point, and this increases sweat activity, although it is seldom visible (but it is palpable – see 'drag' palpation discussed below) (Simons et al 1999, Lewit 1999).
5. There may be loss of hair in target areas (e.g. in the lower limb when there are paraspinal trigger points in the lumbar region) (Gunn 1989).
6. Other skin and fascial changes, as described below, are quite easily palpated, but are seldom visible (Lewit 1999).

Heat, moisture and texture (Simons et al 1999)

- There will usually be altered skin temperature over the trigger point and/or the target zone (increased or decreased) (Fig. 6.1).
- Altered skin humidity (hydrosis, sweat) will be noted over the trigger point and/or the target zone.
- Skin texture changes are common over the trigger point, leading to a rough sandpaper-like quality.

The skill levels required to accurately identify trigger points, and some of the ways of gaining these skills, are summarized in Box 6.1.

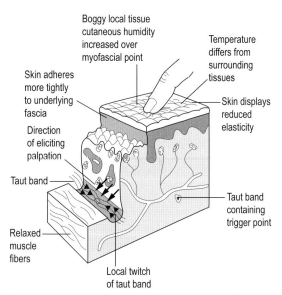

Figure 6.1 Altered physiology of tissues in region of myofascial trigger point. (From Chaitow & DeLany 2000.)

Box 6.1   The skills needed to identify trigger points

Palpation skills require practice before accuracy is reliable. Not surprisingly, research and experience confirms that experienced therapists, who are trained to palpate for tissue changes and landmarks, are more accurate in their findings than those who are not trained adequately (Hsieh et al 2000, Simons et al 1999).

You should be able to identify and name the following by palpation:

- bony structures
- individual muscles (where possible)
- tendons and ligaments, as well as palpable thickenings, bands and nodules within the myofascial tissues.

If you cannot palpate these accurately, then regular practice will help develop and refine your ability.

Useful exercises to develop these skills will be found in the book *Palpation and Assessment Skills* (Chaitow 1996).

To work with trigger points it is also important to have a good knowledge of the fiber arrangement of different muscles. This will allow you to obtain more accurate and reliable results.

Knowledge of (or accessible charts showing) trigger point reference zones (such as the maps in Chapter 4) are helpful until the locations of the major trigger points in the body have been memorized.

As we have seen, the important features of trigger points, as defined by Simons et al (1999), include:

1. a taut palpable band
2. the presence of an extremely painful nodule lying in the taut band
3. a recognizable referral pattern (usually pain) when pressure is applied to the nodule (active with familiar referral, latent with unfamiliar referral)
4. a painful limit to full stretch of the muscle.

Developing skills for trigger point palpation

Central trigger points are usually palpable either with flat palpation (against underlying structures) or with pincer compression (tissue held between thumb and fingers) (Figs 6.2 and 6.3).

Neuromuscular therapy assessment involves a variety of different palpation strategies, using fingers and thumbs as a rule (Figs 6.4 and 6.5).

The fiber arrangement of all muscle tissues should be considered when palpating. It is also possible for the soft tissues to be carefully rolled between fingers and thumb to assess quality, density, fluidity and other characteristics that may offer information about the state of the muscle (e.g. is it fibrous, tense, swollen?).

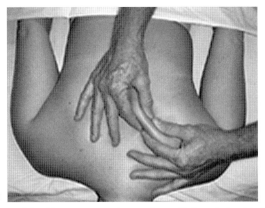

(A)

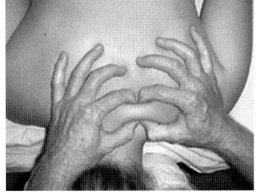

(B)

Figure 6.2   Pincer compression may be applied precisely with the fingertips or with finger pads for a more general release. (From Chaitow & DeLany 2000.)

Box 6.1 The skills needed to identify trigger points – *cont'd*

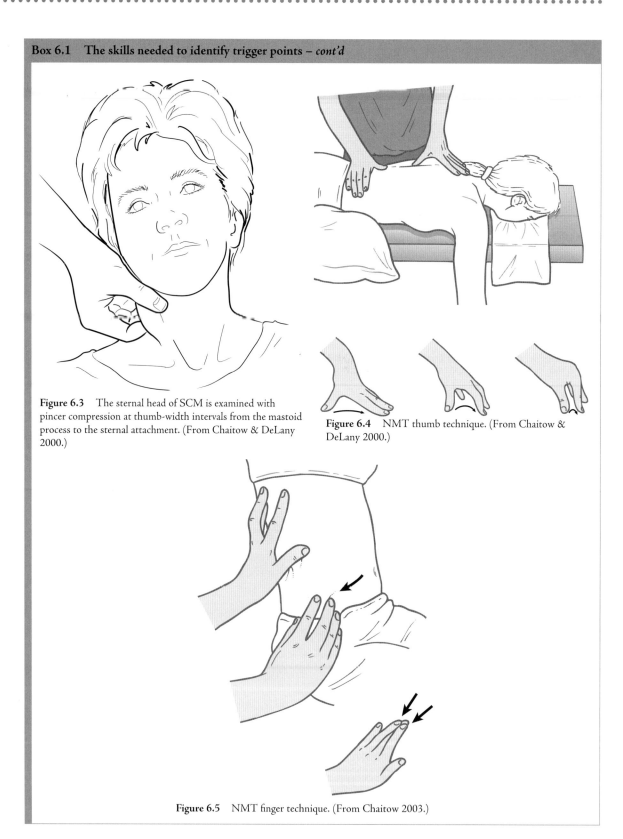

Figure 6.3 The sternal head of SCM is examined with pincer compression at thumb-width intervals from the mastoid process to the sternal attachment. (From Chaitow & DeLany 2000.)

Figure 6.4 NMT thumb technique. (From Chaitow & DeLany 2000.)

Figure 6.5 NMT finger technique. (From Chaitow 2003.)

LOCATING TRIGGER POINTS

Remember that the identification of an active trigger point, central or attachment, relies on finding a local tender spot ('nodule'), lying in a taut muscle band, that reproduces recognizable symptoms when pressed.

1. It is often useful to perform an 'off-body scan' (manual thermal diagnosis), as described in Box 6.2. This method gives evidence of variations in local circulation, probably resulting from differences in tone, and possibly of inflammation and/or ischemia. Trigger point activity is likeliest in areas of greatest 'difference' (temperature contrast) noted when scanning.
2. Movement of skin on fascia – resistance to easy gliding of skin on fascia indicates the general location of reflex activity, i.e. possible trigger point (Lewit 1999), and can indicate lymphatic congestion which may be contributing to the problem (Box 6.3).
3. There will be a local loss of skin elasticity – and this can refine localization of the site of trigger points. Palpation for skin elasticity is described in Box 6.4.
4. Extremely light single-digit stroking ('skin-on-skin'), which seeks to locate a 'drag' sensation (evidence of increased hydrosis, in and under the skin), which offers pinpoint accuracy of location. Drag palpation methods are described in Box 6.5.
5. Digital pressure (angled rather than perpendicular) into the suspected tissues seeks confirmation of active trigger or latent trigger points (Kuchera & McPartland 1997). See Figure 6.11.

Boxes 6.1 to 6.5 describe the skills needed to use skin palpation to identify trigger points.

An exercise is outlined below to help you to discover which of these methods is best suited to your work.

Certainly it is not practical to perform all these methods on each patient in each area suspected of trigger point activity.

You need to evaluate which of these works best for you.

It is suggested that you attempt an assessment in which you compare the reliability and accuracy of all these methods, with each other, on one individual.

Have someone lie prone:

1. Perform an off-body scan for temperature variations (remembering that cold may suggest ischemia, hot may indicate irritation/inflammation). Note areas that are 'different'.
2. Now palpate directly for thermal (heat) variations by molding your hands lightly to the tissues, to assess for temperature differences.

3. Avoid lengthy hand contact or you will change the status of whatever you are palpating. A few seconds should be adequate.
4. Pay particular attention to those 'different' areas (comparing one area with another, and also comparing the 'touch' palpation with the scan palpation), and evaluate skin adherence to underlying fascia, using light 'pushing' of assessed structures, and/or skin rolling, and/or tissue-lifting methods.
5. Ask yourself whether such areas correspond with information gained from the scanning and thermal palpation assessments.
6. Using those areas where dysfunction has been indicated by previous assessments (1 to 5 above), look for variations in local skin elasticity (Lewit's 'skin stretch').
7. Reduced elastic quality indicates a possible hyperalgesic ('very sensitive') zone and probable deeper dysfunction (e.g. trigger point) or pathology.
8. Finally attempt to identify reflexively active areas (trigger points, etc.) by means of very light single-digit palpation, seeking the phenomenon of 'drag'.
9. Do these findings agree with each other? They should, or at least some of them should.
10. Which was the most efficient way of identifying trigger points for you.

NEUROMUSCULAR TECHNIQUES (NMT)

Neuromuscular techniques include a variety of soft tissue methods, often massage based. These are briefly described below. Compression is one of the main NMT methods used to deactivate trigger points, although a number of massage strokes are used, in different ways and sequences.

More detail of NMT procedures will be found in the following texts:

- Chaitow L, DeLany J 2000 *Clinical Applications of Neuromuscular Techniques*, Volume 1, *Upper Body*. Churchill Livingstone
- Chaitow L, DeLany J 2002 *Clinical Applications of Neuromuscular Techniques*, Volume 2, *Lower Body*. Churchill Livingstone
- Chaitow L 2003 *Modern Neuromuscular Techniques*. 2nd edition. Churchill Livingstone.

European NMT uses a variety of thumb and finger strokes to search the body tissues for dysfunctional areas, including trigger points.

An example of the sequence of strokes used in European (also known as Lief's) NMT is shown in

Box 6.2   Thermography in bodywork

Various forms of thermal assessment are being used to identify trigger point activity and other forms of dysfunction, including infrared, electrical and liquid crystal methods (Baldry 1993), as well as manual thermal diagnosis (MTD) (Barrell 1997).

Swerdlow & Dieter (1992) found, after examining 365 patients with demonstrable trigger points in the upper back, that:

> Although thermographic 'hot-spots' are present in the majority, these sites are not necessarily where the trigger points are located.

It is just as likely for trigger points to lie in ischemic, fibrotic tissue that would scan (or feel) 'cold'.

Thermal examination of the reference zone (target area), to which a trigger point refers or radiates, usually shows skin temperature to be raised, but not always (Simons 1993).

Scanning

Scanning the skin surface by hand helps to establish areas which apparently differ from each other in temperature.

French osteopath Jean-Pierre Barrell has established that areas which scan (non-touching) as 'hot' are only truly warmer/hotter than surrounding areas in 75% of instances (Barrell 1997).

Apparently when scanning manually for heat, any area that is markedly different from surrounding tissues, in temperature terms, is considered 'hot' by the brain.

Manual scanning for heat is therefore an accurate way of assessing 'difference' between tissues but not their actual thermal status.

1. Stand at waist level, with your palpation patient prone on the treatment table, exposed from the waist up.
2. Hold your dominant hand, with palm down, close to the surface of the back (about 1 to 2 inches/2.5 to 5 cm).
3. Make steady, deliberate sweeps of the hand to and fro, across the back, until all of it has been scanned.
4. Keep the hand moving slowly because if it remains still, or moves too slowly, you have nothing to compare, and if you move too fast, you will not register the slight changes as the hand passes from one area to another.
5. Approximately 4–5 inches (10–15 cm) should be scanned per second.
6. Different aspects and areas of the hand may be more sensitive than others. Test whether your sensitivity is greater in the palm, near the wrist, or on the dorsum of the hand, as you evaluate areas that feel warmer or cooler than others.

Having identified areas that scan as different from each other, and having charted these on an outline of the human body, it is useful to actually feel the skin to see whether what scanned as 'hot' or 'cold' actually *feels* different when you touch it.

Choose an area or two of the skin that scanned as the most obviously different from surrounding skin.

Place your hand (palm) or finger pads onto this for a few seconds, and then onto surrounding skin, and see whether it actually feels different (hotter or colder).

You may be able to confirm a difference, but this is not always possible, for reasons outlined in Figure 6.6.

This explains that the accuracy of thermal evaluation, when you are touching the patient's skin, depends on a great many variables, including your own levels of sweat activity and that of the patient, as well as rate of blood flow through the tissues (yours and the patient's), and the thickness of skin and whether or not there are materials (oil, tissue debris, etc.) between the two skin surfaces (Adams et al 1982).

Scanning may be more accurate than actual touching of tissues when attempting to evaluate differences.

Chart what you find, and test these more precisely with manual palpation, using one of the 'skin assessment' methods described in this chapter.

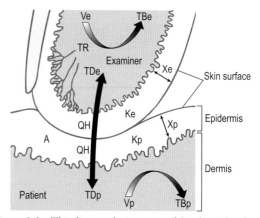

Figure 6.6   This diagram depicts some of the physical and physiologic factors that affect the thermoreceptor (TR) discharge rate and consequently the temperature sensed in an examiner's skin in contact with a patient's skin. The temperature and its rate of change of the examiner's thermoreceptor are functions of the net effects of the time that the tissues are in contact, their contact area (A), the temperatures (TBe and TBp) and volume flow rates (Ve and Vp) of blood perfusing the examiner's and patient's skin, epidermal thickness (Xe and Xp) and thermal conductivity (Ke and Kp) of both, dermal temperature (TDe and TDp) of both, as well as of the net heat exchange rate (QH) between the two tissues. QH is strongly affected by the heat transfer properties of material trapped between the two skin surfaces, for example air, water, oil, grease, hand lotion, dirt, tissue debris, fabric (Adams et al 1982). (From Chaitow 1996.)

Box 6.3   Palpation method based on German connective tissue massage (*Bindegewebsmassage*) (Dicke 1978)

- The patient should be seated or lying prone (Fig. 6.7).
- Both hands are applied flat in order to displace (slide) the skin and subcutaneous tissues against the fascia, with small to-and-fro pushes.
- The amount of movement (slide) possible depends on tension of the tissues and on what is happening in deeper tissues.
- When trigger points (or major dysfunction) exist in the deeper muscle the amount of sliding possible, of skin on fascia, will be reduced (Bischof & Elmiger 1960).
- With your fingers lightly flexed and using only enough pressure to produce adherence between the fingertips and the skin (do not slide on the skin, instead slide the skin on the underlying fascia), make a series of short pushing motions, at the same time, with both hands.
- Ease the tissues (skin on fascia) to the elastic barrier on each side.
- Pay particular attention to comparing areas where 'difference' (heat or cold) was sensed during the scan exercise.

- The pattern of testing is usually performed from inferior to superior, either moving the tissues superiorly or bilaterally, in an obliquely diagonal direction toward the spine.
- Whether your patient is prone or seated, tissues from the buttocks to the shoulders can be tested, always comparing the sides for symmetry of range of movement of the skin, sliding to its elastic barrier.
- Try to identify local areas where your 'push' of skin on fascia reveals restriction as compared with its opposite side.
- It is also useful to gently lift a skinfold from the fascia (Fig. 6.8) looking for differences compared to surrounding tissues.

Compare the findings using this method with those achieved by 'skin on fascia pushes' as described above.

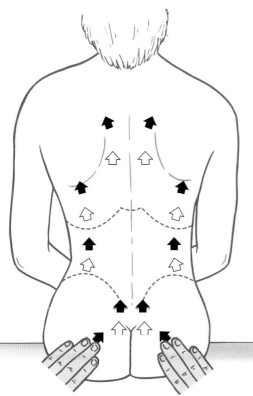

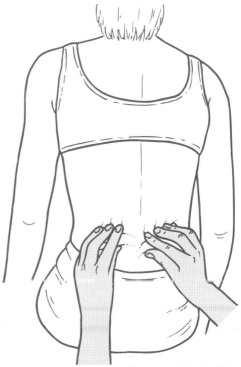

Figure 6.7   Testing tissue mobility by bilaterally 'pushing' skin with finger pads. (From Chaitow 1996.)

Figure 6.8   Assessing bilateral elasticity of skin by lifting it in folds or 'rolling' it. (From Chaitow 1996.)

Box 6.4   Skin elasticity assessment

Lewit & Olsanska (2004) have developed a painless and very effective skin stretching diagnostic and treatment method. The assessment method is described below, and the treatment approach in Chapter 7.

- The skin is stretched, with a minimum of force, to take up the slack.
- At its end-position a slight 'springiness' should still be felt.
- A series of similar stretches are performed, in various directions, over the area being assessed (e.g. where a scan indicated a 'difference' – see Box 6.2).
- Areas of skin that lie over trigger points called hyperalgesic skin zones (HSZ) by Lewit (simply meaning that they are more sensitive than surrounding tissues).
- The skin in these zones will offer a 'stiff' resistance after the elastic slack is taken up, compared with normal skin (which has a springiness even at the end of range).

Apples and oranges

We should only compare like with like, not apples with oranges.

It is important to only compare the quality of skin elasticity in one area with skin in that same area, and not with skin in quite different areas.

For example, skin overlaying the lumbar paraspinal muscles should not be compared with skin overlaying the thoracic paraspinal muscles.

The first would usually be relatively 'loose', and the other fairly 'tight', as a natural matter of course.

However, if one area of thoracic paraspinal skin elasticity is compared with another area of thoracic paraspinal skin elasticity, and one of these is much less elastic than the other, this is evidence that reflex activity (facilitation or trigger points) may exist below the 'tight' skin area.

At first, it is necessary to practice this method slowly. Eventually it should be possible to move fairly rapidly over an area which is being searched for evidence of reflex activity.

Method

- Your patient should be lying prone.
- Choose an area to be assessed that was 'different' on scanning, and that also showed an abnormal degree of skin-on-fascia adherence (see Box 6.3).
- Place your two index fingers right next to each other, on the skin, side by side or pointing towards each other, with no pressure at all onto the skin, just a contact touch (Fig. 6.9A).
- Lightly and slowly separate your fingers, feeling the skin stretch as you do so (Fig. 6.9B).
- Take the stretch to its 'easy' limit without forcibly stretching the skin, just to the point where resistance is first felt.
- This is the 'barrier of resistance'.
- Now, with a little more effort, 'spring' the skin further apart, to its absolute elastic limit.
- Release this stretch and move both fingers 0.5 cm (quarter of an inch) to one side of this first position, and test again, in the same way, and in the same direction of pull, separating the fingers.
- Perform exactly the same sequence over and over again until the entire area of tissue has been searched.
- Try to make sure that the rhythm you adopt is not too slow or to fast – it is suggested that one stretch per second be performed.
- If you sense that the skin is not as elastic as it was on the previous stretch you may have identified a hyperalgesic skin zone (HSZ).
- By applying either finger or thumb pressure to the center of that small zone, you may be able to feel the taut band and its nodular center.
- After sustained pressure on this for 3 to 5 seconds, the patient may report radiating symptoms to a distant site (meaning that you are pressing on a trigger point).
- Your question will be to ask whether the pain is familiar, a part of the symptoms you are attempting to eliminate.

Box 6.4   Skin elasticity assessment – *cont'd*

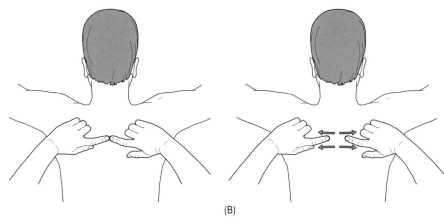

(A)   (B)

Figure 6.9   A: Fingers touch each other directly over skin to be tested – very light skin contact only. B: Pull apart to assess degree of skin elasticity – compare with neighboring skin area. (From Chaitow 1996.)

Box 6.5   Drag palpation (Lewit 1999)

It is possible to assess the skin for variations in skin friction by lightly running a fingertip across the skin surface (no lubricant should be used).

If you are even slightly confused as to what it is that you are trying to feel, remove a watch or bracelet (or have someone else remove their watch or bracelet) and lightly run a finger across the skin that was under the strap, as well as over the adjacent skin.

By running your palpating finger(s) over both 'dry' and 'moist' skin, you should easily be able to feel the difference in drag, friction and resistance.

This palpation method can be used to compare areas that scanned or palpated as 'different' from surrounding tissues, or to rapidly investigate any local area for trigger point activity.

- The degree of pressure required is minimal – skin touching skin is all that is necessary – a 'feather-light touch' (Fig. 6.10).
- Movement of a single palpating digit (pad of the index or middle finger is best) should be purposeful, not too slow and certainly not very rapid. Around 3–5 cm (1–2 inches) per second is a satisfactory speed (if you move too slowly you will not easily pick up differences, and if you move too fast you will miss the information that is waiting for you).
- Feel for any sense of 'drag', which suggests a resistance to the easy, smooth passage of the finger across the skin surface.
- A sense of 'dryness', 'sandpaper', a slightly harsh or rough texture, may all indicate increased presence of sweat on, or increased fluid in, the tissues.

The method of drag palpation is extremely accurate and speedy. It identifies increased sympathetic activity in the tissues, manifested by sweat.

A trigger point will commonly be found below such findings.

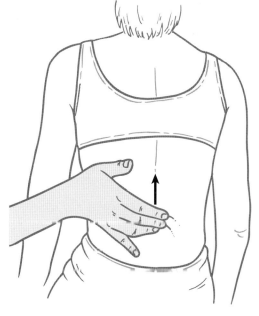

Figure 6.10   Assessing variations in skin friction (drag, resistance). (From Chaitow 1996.)

Figures 6.12 and 6.13. These illustrate brief examples of a comprehensive evaluation that searches (assesses) the body for local dysfunction, before treatment starts.

NMT assessment (finger and thumb) strokes are used in treatment by increasing the degree of pressure applied, in very much the same way as that described in the Thai massage method discussed in Chapter 7, using body weight. See Figure 6.12C.

How much pressure is used in NMT assessment, and how much in NMT treatment?

The various pressures needed to test a possible trigger point for pain were outlined in Chapter 5. The same approach is expanded on below.

If you touch the skin, with no pressure, just 'skin-on-skin', you will not be pressing into the tissues at all.

This is the level of pressure to use when performing 'drag' palpation, as described in this chapter, or to assess thermal (heat/cold) status, as discussed in Box 6.2.

If you press into the tissues sufficiently to have a sense that there is a degree of pressure back against your finger, thumb or hand, you will have reached what has been called the 'rejection' level – where the tissues are resisting (Pick 1999).

About halfway between touch, and the rejection level, is what can be called the 'working level'.

This is the level where your sense of tissue change will be keenest. This gives you an ability to distinguish normal from abnormal tissue (hypertonic, fibrotic, edematous, etc.).

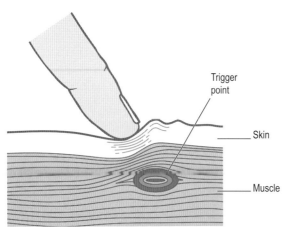

Figure 6.11 Trigger points are areas of local facilitation that can be housed in any soft tissue structure, most usually muscle and/or fascia. Palpation from the skin or at depth may be required to localize them. (From Chaitow 2003.)

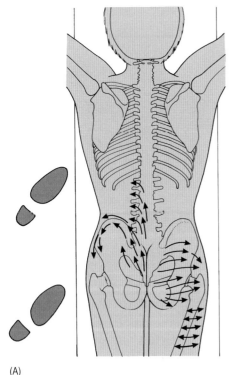 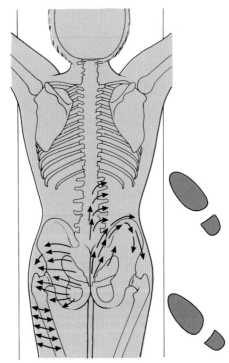

Figure 6.12A and B
Positions in the pelvis/hip region for application of NMT.

(A) (B)

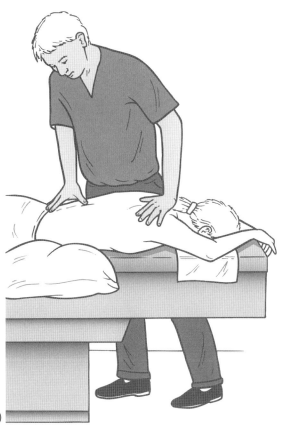

(C)

Figure 6.12C NMT – practitioner's posture should ensure a straight treating arm for ease of transmission of body weight, as well as leg positions that allow for the easy transfer of weight and center of gravity. These postures assist in reducing energy expenditure and ease spinal stress. (From Chaitow 2003.)

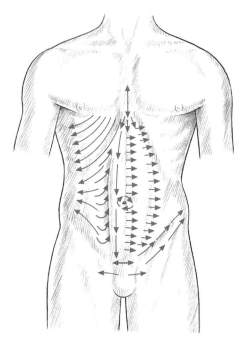

Figure 6.13 Neuromuscular abdominal technique. Suggested lines of application to access primary trigger point and attachment sites, and interfaces between different muscle groups. Note that the lines of application on this chart show one side only, and a full assessment/treatment involves these thumb or finger strokes being applied on each side of the body. (From Chaitow 2003.)

And this is the amount of pressure that is recommended in NMT – where you will be 'meeting and matching' tissue tension.

Depending upon whether you are attempting to apply this pressure to tense muscle, or soft relaxed muscle, the amount of pressure will change. You will also use very different amounts of pressure when you attempt to palpate the soft tissues of the head (overlying bone) and when you are palpating abdominal soft tissues that overlie soft organs.

So finding the 'working level' requires a *variable pressure*, which will not be the same in different parts of the body, and on different tissues, offering different degrees of tension and resistance.

When you are treating dysfunction you will usually be working at 'rejection' level, when you are trying to compress, friction or stretch tissues.

The aim should be to be able to switch from touch, to working, to rejection levels, and back again, as the

tissue status changes, and depending on what it is you want to achieve – to feel? to assess? to treat?

American version NMT uses basic massage strokes, particularly gliding ones, to evaluate for and treat trigger points (Fig. 6.14) and also uses a wooden, rubber-tipped instrument ('T-Bar') to minimize stress on the thumbs and fingers (Fig. 6.15).

Both European and American NMT methods also use compression and a variety of positional release and stretching methods to deactivate trigger points.

In Chapter 7 (Box 7.9) there is a description of traditional Thai massage (TTM) applied to myofascial (trigger point) pain. Although applied in a different sequence to NMT, there seem to be strong similarities. This should not be surprising because European NMT originally derived from a 'Westernization', by osteopaths and chiropractors Stanley Lief and Boris Chaitow, of a traditional Indian (Ayurvedic) massage approach, back in the 1930s.

A sequence known as integrated neuromuscular inhibition technique (described in Chapter 7, Box 7.6) offers a sensitive selection of methods that both locate and deactivate triggers.

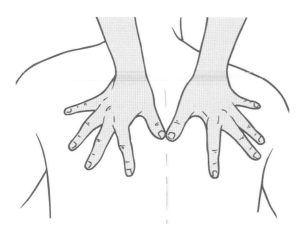

Figure 6.14 The fingers lead and steady the thumbs, which are the primary tools used in most of the gliding techniques. (From Chaitow 2003.)

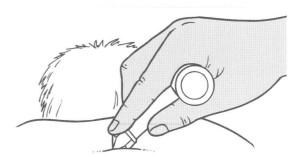

Figure 6.15 A beveled-tip pressure bar may be used in grooves and under bony ledges not easily reached with the thumbs, such as here in the spinal lamina groove. (From Chaitow 2003.)

HEAD AND FACE PAIN PATIENTS

Let's return to the case of the person we discussed earlier in this chapter, with face and head pain (and possibly other symptoms such as increased nasal and sinus secretions), whose trigger points you are searching for in upper trapezius and sternomastoid muscles.

The description in Box 6.6 of NMT evaluation (American version) of upper trapezius is taken from Chaitow & DeLany (2000, Chapter 11).

RSI – REPETITIVE STRAIN INJURY

A brief note is offered in Box 6.7 regarding palpation for trigger points related to repetitive strain problems.

PALPATING SCARS

Lewit & Olsanska (2004) describe what to look for when palpating for trigger points close to scar tissue.

> The characteristic findings on the skin are increased skin drag, owing to increased moisture (sweating); skin stretch will be impaired and the skin fold will be thicker. If the scar covers a wider area, it may adhere to the underlying tissues, most frequently to bone. In the abdominal cavity, we meet resistance in some direction, which is painful. Just as with other soft tissue, after engaging the barrier and waiting, we obtain release after a short latency, almost without increasing pressure. This can be of great diagnostic value, because if, after engaging the barrier the resistance does not change, this is not due to the scar but to some intra-abdominal pathology.

See Figure 7.34 in Chapter 7 for an illustration of this method.

Lewit & Olsanska (2004) point out that not all layers of a scar may be 'active', and that it is important to examine all layers, as part of the assessment.

It is useful to remember that for cosmetic reasons, during surgery, the skin is cut where it is less likely to be seen. The actual operation is, however, carried out in deeper layers, and often at a distance from where the skin was cut. It is in the scar tissue, in the deeper layers, that painful areas may be found, and these should be treated.

After locating an active scar (pain is produced by stretching the tissues around the scar), the question is whether the scar relates to the patient's condition – whether or not it is 'active', and whether or not the patient recognizes the painful symptoms as being familiar.

Treatment of scar trigger points is discussed in Chapter 7.

OTHER WAYS OF IDENTIFYING TRIGGER POINTS

1. Measuring skin resistance to electricity is a way of localizing the same areas that would be identified by 'drag' palpation (described in Box 6.5), and many acupuncturists (and others) use small machines to do this. Resistance to a mild electric current passing through the skin will be reduced when there is moisture (sweat) in or on the skin – and this is precisely what you will be palpating using drag palpation. The extra moisture is due to

(*List continues on p. 87*)

Box 6.6   American version NMT assessment of upper trapezius

- The patient lies supine.
- To assess the cervical portion of upper trapezius the fibers of upper trapezius are targeted (Fig. 6.16).
- These lie directly beside the spinous processes, running vertically up the back and sides of the neck before turning laterally near the base of the neck, running toward the shoulder.
- With no lubrication at this stage these fibers can easily be grasped between the thumb and fingers and compressed, one side at a time or both sides simultaneously, at thumb-width intervals the length of the cervical region.
- If the head is in slight extension this softens the tissues, making grasping them easier.
- The occipital attachment of upper trapezius can be examined using light finger friction, searching for nodules and bands of tension.
- The patient's arm, on the side being worked on, should be placed on the table with the elbow bent and upper arm abducted in order to reduce tension in the muscle.
- The center of the upper portion of the upper trapezius should be grasped and the fibers held between thumb and two or three fingers (Fig. 6.17A).
- A similar pressure could also be applied to trigger points in sternomastoid (Fig. 6.17B).
- Pincer pressure should be applied in this way, to thumb-width segments, along the full length of the upper fibers of the muscle, to examine them for the presence of trigger points.
- It is useful to drag two or three fingers along the anterior surface of the muscle, while at the same time the thumb provides counter-pressure from the posterior aspect of the muscle.
- As the fingers run across the hidden deep fibers, palpable bands and trigger point nodules may be felt.
- A static pincer compression may be applied to any taut bands or nodule discovered in this way, to see if

the pain that results refers or radiates, and whether the pain is familiar to the patient.
- Recent research has shown that this type of simple applied pressure is enough to reduce trigger point activity, even if nothing else is done (Fryer & Hodgson 2005).

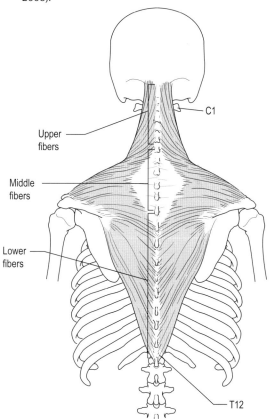

Figure 6.16   Posterior view of trapezius indicating upper, middle and lower portions. (From Chaitow & DeLany 2000.)

Figure 6.17   A: The outermost fibers of upper trapezius may be rolled between the thumb and fingers to identify taut bands. Elevation of the elbow of the treating hand may reduce strain on the wrist which may be indicated in this illustration. (From Chaitow & DeLany 2000.)

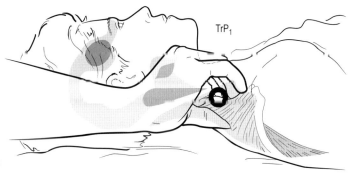

(A)

Box 6.6   American version NMT assessment of upper trapezius – *cont'd*

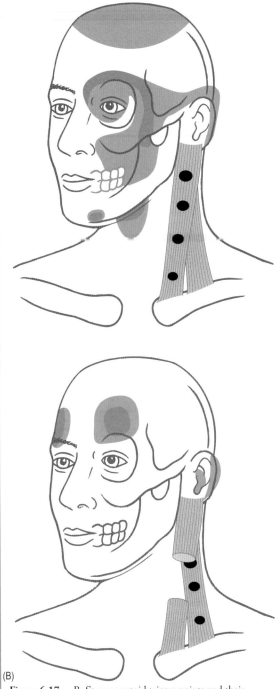

(B)

Figure 6.17   B: Sternomastoid trigger points and their referral points. (From Chaitow & DeLany 2000.)

- Toothpick-sized strands of tense tissue in the upper trapezius often produce extremely painful referrals into the face and eyes.
- The practitioner should be seated at the head of the table with the thumb placed at approximately the mid-fiber level.
- From there it is possible to glide laterally toward the acromioclavicular joint (Fig. 6.18).
- This gliding motion is repeated several times, feeling for anything deep in the muscle that is taut, nodular or uncomfortable.
- The thumb is then returned to the middle of the muscle belly and the glide is performed toward the spine.
- This should be repeated several times.
- These alternating, gliding techniques may be repeated several times from the muscle's center (belly) toward its attachment sites.
- These actions allow for assessment, and because it also spreads the shortened sarcomeres it will help to elongate any taut bands that may be present.
- A double-thumb glide can also be applied by spreading the fibers from the center simultaneously toward the two ends – this can be thought of as involving both assessment and treatment at the same time (Fig. 6.19).
- Central trigger points in these upper fibers refer strongly into the head, and particularly into the eye.
- Attachment trigger points and tenderness may be associated with tension from central trigger points, and may not respond well until central trigger points have been deactivated (see Chapter 7).
- Upper trapezius attachments should receive static pressure from the finger or thumb in order to establish whether previously active attachment points have been eased by the gliding strokes on the central fibers.
- Thumb pressure should be angled anteriorly against the trapezius attachment on the clavicle so that static pressure can be applied (Fig. 6.20).
- Care is needed that pressure is not applied more medially than a few finger widths from the acromioclavicular joint, as the brachial plexus lies deep to the clavicle. Deep pressure here can irritate nerves and accompanying blood vessels.

Following these deep assessment compressions and glides, lubricated, gliding strokes may be used to soothe the tissues.

Alternative

An alternative NMT approach, using Lief's European NMT,

Box 6.6   American version NMT assessment of upper trapezius – *cont'd*

would follow specific directions of thumb and finger stroke in order to achieve a similar result to that outlined above. This would access triggers in both sternomastoid and upper trapezius. The 'map' of these strokes is shown in Figure 6.21.

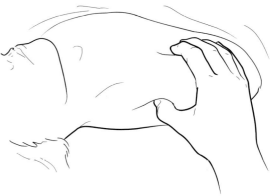

Figure 6.20   Pressure or friction to the clavicular attachment of trapezius is carefully applied to assess tenderness due to inflammation, which is often associated with attachment trigger points. (From Chaitow & DeLany 2000.)

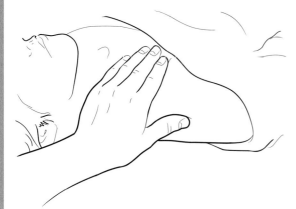

Figure 6.18   The upper trapezius fibers may be pressed against the underlying supraspinatus with gliding strokes in lateral or medial directions. (From Chaitow & DeLany 2000.)

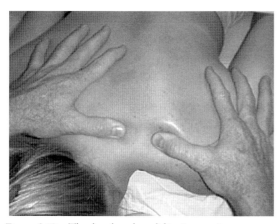

Figure 6.19   The thumbs, when gliding in opposite directions, provide precise traction of the fibers and a local myofascial release. (From Chaitow & DeLany 2000.)

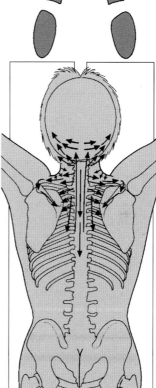

Figure 6.21   Lief's NMT 'map' for cervical and upper thoracic areas. (From Chaitow & DeLany 2000.)

Box 6.7   Repetitive strain injury (RSI)

In conditions such as repetitive strain injury, for example affecting the elbow, arm or wrist, palpation should take the form of gentle probing of the known sites (Figs 6.22, 6.23 and 6.24). Trigger points contribute greatly to RSI-related pain.

With RSI there may also be active inflammation, so care is needed in applying pressure – see cautions earlier in this chapter.

By using all or any of the assessment methods listed above (skin palpation, NMT, etc.) or by carefully feeling through the tissues near the bellies of the muscles of the region, areas of tightness, contracture and pain may be found. Direct sustained pressure for several seconds may then result in the patient reporting a 'familiar' pain. You will have identified a source of the problem. In cases of RSI, manual treatment is only part of the rehabilitation

process. Changing the ways the person is using and possibly abusing the tissues (posture, ergonomics, etc.) is equally important. But without deactivation of the *sources* of the pain – the active trigger points – it will be more difficult to get the person to change the habits that are the *cause* of the pain.

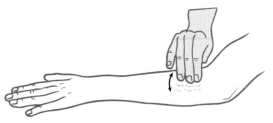

Figure 6.22   Probing for trigger points.

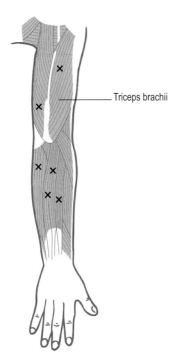

Figure 6.23   Trigger point sites triceps brachii.

Triceps brachii

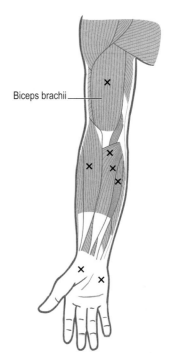

Figure 6.24   Trigger point sites biceps brachii.

Biceps brachii

sympathetic nervous system activity, something that is a key part of the trigger point evolution.

2. Some clinics and practitioners use thermal imaging to localize 'hot' and 'cold' spots that are likely to house trigger points. This is useful in research studies or a photographic record of changes resulting from treatment, and undoubtedly provides objective evidence of 'difference' from surrounding tissue. Skilled 'off the body scanning' (as described earlier in this chapter) can usually gather the same information without the high-tech machinery needed.

3. Use of ultrasound has been promoted for trigger point diagnosis. However, research does not support the validity of this method. Eleven patients with identified active trigger points were assessed using diagnostic ultrasound on both the trigger point side and the non-trigger point side of the body. The results showed that the method was not particularly accurate in identifying the trigger points (Lewis & Tehan 1999).

CLINICAL NOTE

Key points from Chapter 6

1. You may discover trigger points while performing a massage.

2. A more efficient way of locating trigger points is to use the pain referral pattern (or symptom picture – such as irritated sinuses from sternomastoid triggers – see Fig. 6.17B) to guide you to the correct muscles to search.

3. Trigger points sometimes create visible changes in the skin (orange peel appearance, for example), making finding them easier.

4. Trigger points change the temperature of the area in which they are located, and in target tissue, making scanning off-the-body a useful part of assessment.

5. Trigger points change the function of skin in their locality, making the skin less elastic and more adherent to underlying structures. This is useful for palpation assessment.

6. Trigger points almost always increase hydrosis (sweat) in skin above them, allowing drag palpation to be a useful tool.

7. Scar palpation is an important part of assessment.

8. Although they are usually safe there are a number of important cautions and contraindications to using deep pressure methods.

9. Neuromuscular technique (NMT) is a useful assessment and treatment approach. There are two versions, European (Lief's) and American.

10. Palpation skills need to be refined to easily identify trigger points unless methods such as electrical skin resistance measurement, or thermal imaging, are being used.

References

Adams T, Steinmetz J, Heisey R et al 1982 Physiological basis for skin properties in palpatory physical diagnosis. Journal of American Osteopathic Association 81(7):441

Baldry P 1993 Acupuncture, trigger points and musculoskeletal pain. Churchill Livingstone, Edinburgh

Barell J-P 1997 Manual thermal diagnosis. Eastland Press, Seattle

Bischof J, Elmiger G 1960 Connective tissue massage: In: Licht E (ed) Massage, manipulation and traction. New Haven, CT

Chaitow L 1996 Palpation and assessment skills. Churchill Livingstone, Edinburgh

Chaitow L 2003 Modern neuromuscular techniques, 2nd edn. Churchill Livingstone, Edinburgh

Chaitow L, DeLany J 2000 Clinical applications of neuromuscular techniques. Vol 1, Upper body. Churchill Livingstone, Edinburgh

de las Peñas C, Campo M, Carnero J et al 2005 Manual therapies in myofascial trigger point treatment: a systematic review. Journal of Bodywork and Movement Therapies 9(1):27–34

Dicke E 1978 A manual of reflexive therapy. Sydney Simons, Scarsdale, New York

Fryer G, Hodgson L 2005 The effect of manual pressure release on myofascial trigger points in the upper trapezius muscle. Journal of Bodywork and Movement Therapies 9(4): in press

Fryer G, Morris T, Gibbons P 2004 Relation between thoracic paraspinal tissues and pressure sensitivity measured by digital algometer. Journal of Osteopathic Medicine 7(2):64–69

Gunn C 1989 Treating myofascial pain. University of Washington, Seattle

Hsieh C Y, Hong C Z, Adams A et al 2000 Interexaminer reliability of the palpation of trigger points in the trunk and lower limb muscles. Archives of Physical Medicine and Rehabilitation 81:258–264

Kuchera M, McPartland J 1997 Myofascial trigger points. In: Ward R (ed) Foundations of osteopathic medicine. Williams & Wilkins, Baltimore

Lewis J, Tehan P 1999 A blinded pilot study investigating the use of diagnostic ultrasound for detecting active myofascial trigger points. Pain 79(l):39–44

Lewit K 1999 Manipulative therapy in rehabilitation of the locomotor system. Butterworths, London

Lewit K, Olsanska S 2004 Clinical importance of active scars: abnormal scars as a cause of myofascial pain. Journal of Manipulative and Physiological Therapeutics 27(6):399–402

Pick M 1999 Cranial sutures. Eastland Press, Seattle

Simons D 1993 Myofascial pain and dysfunction review. Journal of Musculoskeletal Pain 1(2):131

Simons D, Travell J, Simons L 1999 Myofascial pain and dysfunction: the trigger point manual. Vol 1: Upper half of body, 2nd edn. Williams & Wilkins, Baltimore

Swerdlow B, Dieter N 1992 Evaluation of thermography. Pain 48:205–213

CHAPTER SEVEN

How to treat trigger points manually

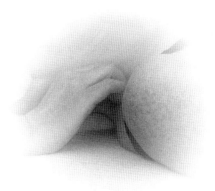

USEFUL TRIGGER POINTS – A REMINDER

Before deciding to treat and deactivate a trigger point you might want to consider whether it could be a useful protective feature, for example in someone who is hypermobile (see Box 1.3 in Chapter 1 for discussion of this possibility).

Trigger points tend to increase tone in the muscles in which they are found, as well as in the muscles to which they refer, and if that increased tone has a supportive stabilizing value, it may be worth considering leaving the trigger points alone until better stabilizing function has been achieved, for example by an appropriate stability and flexibility exercise program, or by use of some form of external support (short-term use of supportive taping, or use of a sacroiliac belt, for example).

ATTENTION TO CAUSES

It is also important for us to remember that every trigger point has a cause (or a variety of causes), and that it is the *underlying* reasons for the trigger point's existence that need to be removed, or changed, if real prevention is to be achieved.

Sometimes of course trigger points do not have a current cause.

They may be the result of past events (such as scar tissue from past surgery or injury – as discussed in Box 7.5 in this chapter).

And sometimes the cause of a trigger point is another trigger point.

To remind yourself about this possibility you may want to revisit the notes on 'key' trigger points, and their satellites in Chapter 3 (see Table 3.1), so that attention is given to the trigger point that may be maintaining more distal points, which will reduce in activity, and sometimes vanish altogether, once the key point has been deactivated.

'IMPOSTER' SYMPTOMS

Pain that looks and feels like musculoskeletal pain, but is actually 'imposter' pain, may represent a more serious pathology. See Chapter 4 for some important examples of these.

This does not mean that trigger points are not commonly also a part of the cause of pain in some painful serious pathological conditions.

What it does mean is that when someone has a life-threatening or well-established, pathology, that person needs comprehensive medical attention, and there is a danger that if pain is modified, for example by trigger point deactivation, focus on other forms of healthcare may be neglected or delayed, with serious consequences.

An example of this might be someone with an underlying cardiovascular problem who develops chest and arm pain due to active trigger points in the scalene muscles.

In such a case, the ideal solution would be for appropriate care to deactivate trigger points, as well as attention from an expert in heart health. Clearly the priority should be given to urging the patient to visit a physician, with trigger point and other manual interventions delayed until a medical diagnosis is available and appropriate medical treatment of the heart condition underway.

Back pain and spinal disease (disc prolapse, tumor, arthritis, etc.), and other forms of pain and neurological dysfunction (neuropathy such as carpal tunnel syndrome, for example) are other examples where myofascial (trigger point) pain may exist alongside more complex causes of pain.

The trigger points need attention, but so do the wider health needs of the patient.

WHAT'S CAUSING OR MAINTAINING THIS TRIGGER?

As well as focusing on offering symptomatic relief by deactivating the trigger points that are responsible for someone's pain, it is also important to have in mind the need to deal with underlying causes of trigger point activity.

Causes and maintaining features can involve overuse, misuse, disuse, trauma, nutritional imbalance, emotional stress – or whatever else might be making adaptive demands. See Chapters 1 and 2 for a reminder of these factors and processes.

Patients need to be informed that while the pain can probably be eased, or removed, through manual treatment, there will be a return of the symptoms, unless the poor posture, stressful work pattern, overuse – or whatever else you have identified as contributing to the problem – is modified or eliminated.

WHAT METHOD?

Once you have decided to deactivate a trigger point that has shown itself to be active, you have various methods to choose from.

NOTE:
1. All the methods outlined below require appropriate training and competence.
2. Most of the methods described in this chapter (apart from manipulation) fall within the scope of practice of all manual (massage) therapists.
3. In Chapter 9 other – non-manual – methods will be described. Whether or not you are licensed to perform the methods discussed in that chapter, it is important to have a good understanding of all of them, as well as of what evidence there is of their possible usefulness. Some of the methods listed in Chapter 9 and in this chapter require specific licensure (acupuncture and dry needling, high-velocity manipulation, for example).

Why should you want to know about methods that lie outside your scope of practice?

Because understanding the methodologies and possible values (and risks) of these non-manual

methods will give you the opportunity to discuss the range of choices knowledgeably and intelligently, with both clients and other healthcare professionals.

Summary

All of the following manual methods and techniques have been shown to be capable of deactivating trigger points, although none of them are always successful (Chaitow & DeLany 2000, Kuchera & McPartland 1997, Simons et al 1999):

1. Inhibitory compression (also called ischemic compression) as used in osteopathic soft tissue manipulation, neuromuscular therapy (NMT), massage and acupressure. This method of applied pressure is now called 'trigger point pressure release' (Simons et al 1999); see Box 7.1.
2. Chilling techniques (vapo-coolant spray or ice), commonly combined with stretching – 'spray and stretch' (Simons et al 1999); see Box 7.2.
3. Positional release methods such as strain/counterstrain (Chaitow & DeLany 2000, Chaitow 2003a, Jones 1981); see Box 7.3.
4. Muscle energy and other stretching techniques, as well as self-help stretching strategies (Chaitow & DeLany 2000, Davies 2001, Simons et al 1999); see Box 7.4.
5. Myofascial release methods (Barnes 1996) and skin myofascial release for scar tissue (Lewit & Olsanka 2004); see Box 7.5.
6. Combination sequences such as integrated neuromuscular inhibition technique (INIT) (Chaitow 1994); see Box 7.6.
7. Correction of associated somatic dysfunction, possibly involving high-velocity thrust (HVT) adjustments and/or osteopathic or chiropractic mobilization methods (Liebenson 1996); see Box 7.7.
8. Manual lymphatic drainage (Foldi & Strossenreuther 2005); see Box 7.8.
9. Massage (de las Peñas 2004); see Box 7.9.
10. Education and correction of contributory and perpetuating factors (posture, diet, stress, breathing habits, etc.) (Bradley 1999); see Box 7.10.

Which treatment method is more effective?

There have been very few attempts to compare different trigger point treatment methods, and this makes it very difficult to be sure which method (if any) is superior to the others.

There is evidence that a combination of methods appears to work more successfully than individual approaches (compression and stretching, for example), although all the trigger point deactivation methods discussed in this chapter have been shown to work on their own, in some cases.

As will be seen in Box 7.1, Hou and colleagues (2002) compared different methods of trigger point treatment, in different combinations:

- ischemic compression
- hot packs plus active range of motion (ROM)
- transcutaneous electric nerve stimulation (TENS)
- spray (cold) and stretch
- interferential current and myofascial release.

Results suggest that compression on its own provides immediate relief, and that combinations of compression with hot packs, active ROM, and/or stretch and spray, and/or myofascial release, add to the benefits.

Comparative study

In another study researchers looked at the immediate benefits of treating an active trigger point in the upper trapezius muscle in different ways.

They compared four commonly used methods as well as a placebo (dummy) treatment (Hong 1994).

The methods they tested were:

1. Ice spray and stretch (Travell & Simons' approach: Simons et al 1999); see Box 7.2.
2. Superficial heat applied by a hydrocollator pack (20–30 minutes).
3. Deep heat applied by ultrasound (1.2–1.5 watt/cm^2 for 5 minutes); see Box 9.6.
4. Dummy ultrasound (0.0 watt/cm^2) as the non-active placebo treatment.
5. Deep pressure soft tissue massage (10–15 minutes of modified connective tissue massage and shiatsu/ischemic compression); see Box 7.1.

Twenty-four patients were selected with active trigger points in their upper trapezius muscles, that had been present for not less than 3 months.

None of these people had received treatment for at least one month before the study.

None of them had any signs of pathology such as nerve disease, disc or degenerative disease.

- The pain threshold of the trigger point area was measured using a pressure algometer three times before treatment and within 2 minutes of treatment. (See Chapter 5 for more on the clinical use of an algometer.)

- The average amount of pressure needed to cause pain was recorded on each occasion.
- A control group were also measured twice (30 minutes apart) but they received no treatment until after the second measurement.

The results showed that *all* methods (but not the placebo ultrasound) produced a significant increase in pain threshold following treatment.

The most significant change in pain levels was found in those patients receiving deep pressure (compression) treatment (as would be used in neuromuscular therapy).

The spray and stretch method was the next most efficient method of achieving increase in pain threshold (which means that after the spray and stretch more pressure was needed to cause pain).

What we learn from these two studies is that:

1. Compression seems to be the most effective method for deactivating trigger points – with light sustained pressure, or intermittent (on-off-on-off) pressure methods usually being superior to very heavy compression (Simons et al 1999).
2. Spray and stretch was the second most effective treatment.
3. Compression, combined with other methods (stretching and/or damp heat, for example) works even better than compression on its own (see Box 7.6 in this chapter for a sequence of integrated deactivation methods – INIT).
4. All these variations are incorporated into neuromuscular technique (or neuromuscular therapy) – NMT.
5. All the methods, except dummy ultrasound, had some beneficial effects.

GUIDELINES FOR CHOOSING POINTS TO TREAT

- What if you locate a great many trigger points in a patient's muscles?
- What if the patient is stressed, in a lot of pain, and feeling fatigued and fragile?
- Are there appropriate guidelines to suggest where to begin, which trigger point to choose for deactivation first?

Fortunately it is possible to make practical suggestions, as to where to begin.

These suggestions are based on the clinical experience of thousands of practitioners who have had to face just these questions, particularly which trigger points should receive attention first (McPartland & Klofat 1995).

1. Choose the area of the body that contains the greatest number of active trigger points.
2. Of the points in that area – say the neck and shoulder region – identify the most painful ones (those that produce the most pain with the least pressure), and of these choose the most medial (nearest the midline), and the most proximal (nearest the head), to treat first.
3. Try to identify key points (see Table 3.1 in Chapter 3), and always select these for treatment first if possible.
4. Key points that are closest to the head (i.e. more proximal) and closest to the midline (i.e. more medial) would be the best to treat first.
5. If you have to choose between central (near the belly) or attachment points, always choose central points for active treatment (see previous chapter for an example of this involving NMT application to upper trapezius trigger points).
6. Attachment points usually ease or deactivate if central points in the same muscle are deactivated.
7. Even in a healthy, robust individual, try to never treat more than five trigger points at any treatment session.
8. The more frail, fatigued, sensitive, elderly (or very young) and pain-ridden the patient, the fewer the number of trigger points that should be treated at any one session (between one and three in such cases) to avoid adaptation overload (see Chapter 2 for discussion of adaptation).
9. Damp heat (hot damp towel, for example) helps ease post-treatment discomfort and speeds recovery after central points have been treated (whatever the method).
10. Ice applications are helpful for attachment points.

LENGTHENING IS IMPORTANT!

Trigger points are self-perpetuating, unless they are treated correctly.

This means that, once symptoms of pain have been relieved (by whatever method), the muscle containing the trigger should be stretched gently to its normal resting length.

Whatever method is used to deactivate a trigger point, whether this involves manual therapy, injection of pharmacological agents such as novocaine or Xylocaine, coolant sprays or acupuncture techniques, there is one essential requirement – that the muscle housing the trigger point should be restored to its normal resting length after, and sometimes during, the treatment.

If this is not done, reactivation of the trigger point is more likely (Simons et al 1999).

Experience suggests that failure to restore the muscle containing the trigger point to its normal resting length will result in the treatment providing only short-term relief.

Whatever stretching methods are used it is important that the process should be gradual, gentle and painless (muscle energy technique and myofascial release are recommended – see Boxes 7.4 and 7.5).

The recommendation of Lewit (1999) and Simons et al (1999) is that muscle energy technique (MET) be used to achieve safe and (relatively) painless stretching.

This calls for gentle isometric contractions followed by stretch (see Boxes 7.4 and 7.5).

Lewit (1999) suggests that, in many instances, simply stretching a muscle – with no other treatment – may be sufficient to deactivate trigger point activity.

Box 7.1   Compression

- Compression techniques are widely used in the treatment of trigger points.
- Compression methods often involve direct finger, thumb (or other) pressure against underlying bone or other soft tissues (Fig. 7.1).
- Precise compression of individual fibers is possible using a pincer palpation, or flat palpation, both of which capture specific bands of tissue for either assessment or treatment purposes.
- Compression can be achieved using a pincer grip, in which flat *finger pad*(s) and thumb grip the tissues lying between them (something like a clothes peg) in order to compress them (Fig. 7.2).
- The *fingertip*(s) can also be used in pincer compression, but they easily slip on tense, taut muscles – such as sternomastoid – causing discomfort.
- A fingertip grip is also more likely to cause microtrauma than use of the flatter pads of the fingers (Fig. 7.3).

Pincer grip – benefits and cautions?

A general thickening in the central portion of a muscle's belly, housing a central trigger point, will usually soften when a broad general pressure is applied, using a flat compression.

Compression may be applied wherever the tissue can be lifted without irritating blood vessels or nerves.

When using any form of compression it is important to pay attention to underlying structures (such as sharp bony surfaces), particularly nerves and blood vessels that might be compressed.

Effects of compression

The following effects are thought to take place during the application of sustained or intermittent digital compression of tissues:

- Ischemia: a cutting off of local circulation until pressure is released, after which a flushing of fresh oxygenated blood occurs (Simons et al 1999).
- 'Neurological inhibition' occurs as a result of a sustained volley of messages to the central nervous system (efferent barrage) (Ward 1997).
- A degree of mechanical stretching occurs, as 'creep' of connective tissue starts (Cantu & Grodin 1992).
- Piezoelectric effects modify the 'gel' (hardened) state of tissues to a more solute ('sol' or softer) state (Barnes 1996).
- Rapid nerve (mechanoreceptor) impulses interfere with slower pain messages and reduce pain messages reaching the brain (this is known as the 'gate theory' because the pain gate is 'closed'; Melzack & Wall 1994) (Fig. 7.4).
- Pain-relieving hormones (endorphins and enkephalins) are released (Baldry 1993).
- Taut bands associated with trigger points release spontaneously when compressed (Simons et al 1999).
- Traditional Chinese medicine suggests modification of energy flow through tissues following pressure application.

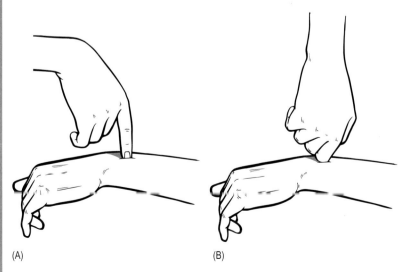

Figure 7.1   A: Finger pressure to test for sensitivity or to treat trigger point on wrist. B: Knuckle pressure to test for sensitivity or to treat trigger point on wrist. (From

(A)   (B)

Box 7.1   Compression – *cont'd*

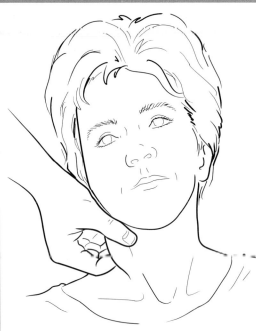

Figure 7.2   The sternal head of sternocleidomastoid is examined with pincer compression at thumb-width intervals from the mastoid process to the sternal attachment. (From Chaitow & DeLany 2000.)

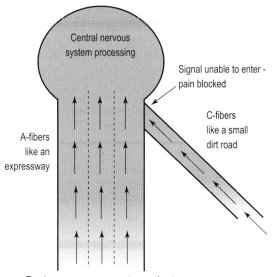

Central nervous system processing

Signal unable to enter - pain blocked

C-fibers like a small dirt road

A-fibers like an expressway

Touch, pressure, movement or moderate acute pain purposefully applied counter irritation which may provide hyperstimulation analgesia.

Figure 7.4   Gate control theory. (Reproduced with permission, from Fritz 1998.)

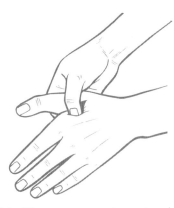

Figure 7.3   Pincer pressure on trigger point at base of thumb. (From Chaitow 2004.)

Box 7.1   Compression – *cont'd*

How firm/deep should compression be?

McPartland (2004) has discussed the change in the method of compression that Simons et al (1999) recommend, compared with that suggested over 20 years ago by Travell & Simons (1983):

> Twenty years ago Travell and Simons treated trigger points with 'ischemic compression' by applying heavy thumb pressure sufficient to produce skin blanching. In the 1999 edition, they recommend applying gentle digital pressure ... that uses the barrier-release concept, in which the finger 'follows' the releasing tissue.

This lighter compression, called 'trigger point pressure release', produces less microtrauma and is less uncomfortable for the patient (and the therapist). If deeper pressure is needed, because of the depth at which a trigger point is located, then an intermittent – 5 seconds on/2 seconds off compression, repeated until a change is perceived or reported, is suggested.

Trigger point deactivation methods in which digital compression is used

Compression method 1
1. Apply firm digital compression to the trigger point sufficient to produce localized discomfort or pain, as well as symptoms in the target area.
2. Maintain this compression for 5 seconds.
3. Release for 2–3 seconds.
4. Reapply pressure (at the same level) and keep repeating, 5 seconds on, 2–3 seconds off, until the patient reports a reduction in local or referred pain, or an increase in pain (which is rare), or until 2 minutes have passed with no change in the pain level.
5. If you were using the integrated neuromuscular inhibition technique (INIT) sequence (see Box 7.6), you would introduce positional release after this initial compression stage (see Box 7.3).

Compression method 2
1. Apply firm digital pressure to the trigger point, sufficient to produce localized discomfort or pain, as well as symptoms in the target area.
2. Maintain the pressure for approximately 10 seconds.
3. Increase the degree of pressure slightly and maintain for a further 10 seconds.
4. Increase the degree of pressure once more and maintain for approximately 10 more seconds.
5. This compression method – as widely used in NMT – seems very similar to the description of traditional Thai massage (TTM) described in Box 7.10. This is not

surprising as NMT (Lief's European version) was derived from traditional Ayurvedic massage methods.
6. Slowly release pressure and, if you are utilizing the INIT sequence (see Box 7.6), you would introduce positional release after this initial compression stage (see Box 7.3).

Compression method 3 (Fryer & Hodgson 2005)
1. This method is similar to method 2, above, but instead of being based on time (10 seconds) it is based on the patient's feedback to you.
2. Compression is applied to a trigger point until localized discomfort, and referred symptoms, are recognized by the patient to represent a score of 7/10, where 10 would be unbearable.
3. The pressure (compression) is maintained until the patient reports a reduction in the pain level (to 5 or less).
4. Pressure is then increased to return the 'score' to 7/10.
5. This is maintained until a further reduction to 5/10 or less is reported by the patient.

What about compression in combination with other methods?

The immediate effect of physical therapeutic modalities on myofascial pain in the upper trapezius muscle was compared in 119 individuals with palpable active myofascial trigger points (Hou et al 2002).

The following methods were compared in various combinations:

- ischemic compression
- hot packs plus active range of motion (ROM)
- transcutaneous electric nerve stimulation
- stretch with spray
- interferential current and myofascial release.

Results suggest that compression on its own provides immediate relief, and that combinations of compression together with hot packs, active ROM, stretch and spray, and/or myofascial release, add to the benefits.

The one certainty that this suggests is that compression should be a major part of treatment that aims to deactivate trigger points.

Self-treatment of trigger points using compression methods?

Self-care is a useful means of empowerment and first aid.

There are a number of books that promote self-assessment and self-treatment of trigger points.

One of the best written, and possibly the most widely available, is *The Trigger Point Therapy Workbook* (Davies 2001). This is highly recommended for home use.

Box 7.1   Compression – *cont'd*

Another useful guide to self-care is *Maintaining Body Balance, Flexibility and Stability* (Chaitow 2004). This book describes self-applied trigger point deactivation (compression, muscle energy, positional release, spray and stretch) as well as a range of rehabilitation and improved breathing approaches. It suggests that home-care advice as given in the book should be used in conjunction with the advice and/or supervision of a licensed practitioner or therapist.

Both the books referenced above (Chaitow 2004, Davies 2001) incorporate use of tools, such as tennis balls (and in the Davies (2001) book, many other types of ball), in order to apply compression to inaccessible areas (Fig. 7.5).

Cautions

There are several important cautions regarding self-applied treatments of any sort, including trigger point deactivation.

1. Underlying causes might be ignored if pain can be relieved, allowing potentially serious conditions to worsen.
2. The amount of pressure and/or stretching might be too enthusiastically applied by someone who has had no training at all, apart from the advice given in a book or magazine article, potentially creating new problems.
3. Too many trigger points might be self-treated at any one time, potentially overloading repair and adaptation potentials. This could exhaust the individual and lead to more pain for a while.

All these cautions and risks apply equally to poorly trained therapists, and are not meant to suggest that self-treatment is not an excellent idea.

Trigger point self-treatment is recommended if:
1. Safety guidelines (how much pressure, how much stretching, how many points at one time, etc.) are followed.
2. Trigger points are only treated once the underlying causes have been recognized, and are being dealt with (better posture, avoidance of overuse, appropriate attention from a healthcare provider, etc.).

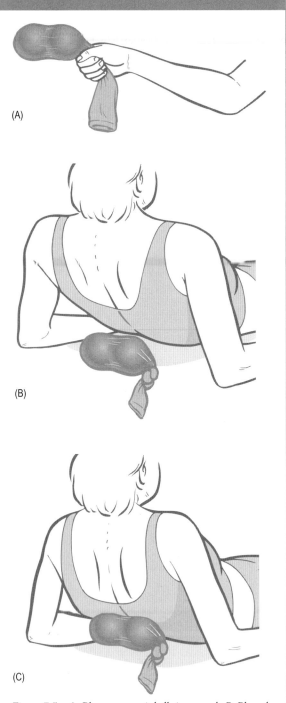

(A)

(B)

(C)

Figure 7.5   A: Place two tennis balls into a sock. B: Place the balls on a carpeted floor. C: Lie so that your spinous processes rest between the balls and the balls press into the tense muscles alongside the spine. (From Chaitow 2004.)

Box 7.2   'Spray and stretch' and other chilling methods

Chilling and stretching a muscle housing a trigger point rapidly assists in its deactivation (Mennell 1974, Travell 1952).

Simons et al (1999) reported that: 'Spray and stretch is the single most effective non-invasive method to inactivate acute trigger points.'

They have also said that the stretch component is the important part of this process, and that the spray is for 'distraction'.

It is important that the coolant spray should be applied *before or during* the stretch, and not *after* the muscle has already been lengthened.

Method

The aim is to chill the surface tissues, while the underlying muscle (housing the trigger point) is being stretched.

- A container is needed of an environmentally friendly vapo-coolant spray (such as 'Gebauer Spray and Stretch') which has a calibrated nozzle that delivers a fine jet stream.
- If this brand cannot be obtained, then fluorimethane is acceptable, and is preferred over ethyl chloride, which is both a health hazard and colder than is needed for this treatment (Simons et al 1999).
- The cold jet stream should be strong enough to carry for at least 3 feet (about 1 meter). (Note that a mist-like spray is less effective.)
- An alternative is to use a cylinder of ice, formed by freezing water in a paper cup and then peeling the cup down to expose the ice edge. A wooden handle can be frozen into the ice to allow for ease of application, as the thin, cold edge of the ice is applied as a series of parallel strokes, running from the trigger point toward the referral zone, while the muscle is at stretch.
- Another method uses a cold drink can that has been partially filled with water and then frozen. The ice-cold metal container can be rolled over the skin during the stretch procedure (in a series, from trigger to target, repetitively).
- Unlike the previous option (edge of ice cylinder) the cold metal can retains its chilling potential, without excessive moisture touching the skin.
- Whichever of these choices you make, the patient should be relaxed and warm.

- If a spray is used, the container should be held 1–2 feet (25 to 50 cm) away from the skin surface, so that the coolant stream meets it at an acute angle, reducing the shock of the impact.
- Each cold sweep should start just proximal to the trigger point (i.e. nearer the head) moving slowly through the reference zone to cover it, and to extend slightly beyond it. (See Figs 7.6 and 7.7.)
- The direction of movement is usually in line with the muscle fibers toward their insertion.
- Both the trigger and reference areas should be chilled because embryonic points may have developed in the referral zone.
- This method deals with both central and attachment trigger points (Simons et al 1999).
- The optimum speed of movement of the sweep/roll over the skin seems to be about 4 inches (10 cm) per second.
- The sweeps are repeated in a rhythm of a few seconds on, and a few seconds off, until all the skin over the trigger and reference areas has been covered once or twice.
- If during the spraying a 'cold pain' develops, or if the application of the spray or ice/canister creates a reference pain, the interval between applications should be lengthened. Take great care not to frost or blanch the skin.
- During the application of cold, or immediately after, the taut fibers should be passively stretched. The fibers should not be stretched before the cold application.
- Steady, gentle, stretching is usually best, maintained for 20–30 seconds.
- After each series of cold applications, active motion is tested. Is movement easier? Is movement less restricted? Is movement less uncomfortable?
- An attempt should be made to restore the full range of motion, but always within the limits of pain, since sudden overstretching can increase existing muscle spasm.
- The entire procedure may occupy 15–20 minutes and should not be rushed.
- Simple home exercises that involve passive or active stretching should be taught to the patient.

Box 7.2   'Spray and stretch' and other chilling methods – *cont'd*

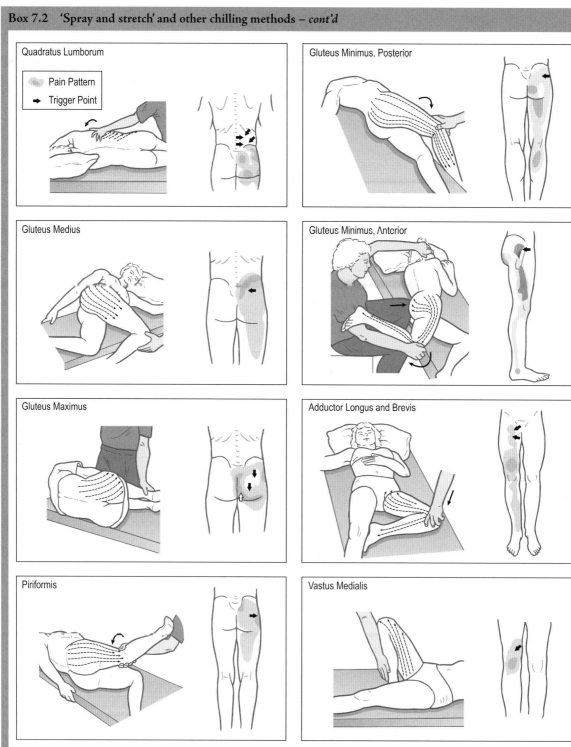

Quadratus Lumborum

Pain Pattern
Trigger Point

Gluteus Minimus, Posterior

Gluteus Medius

Gluteus Minimus, Anterior

Gluteus Maximus

Adductor Longus and Brevis

Piriformis

Vastus Medialis

Figure 7.6   Travell trigger point pain patterns common in patients with gravitational strain pathophysiology (GSP). Local treatment with vapo-coolant spray and stretch technique requires postural alignment and systemic integrating techniques to avoid recurrence. (Adapted with permission from Simons 1987.)

Box 7.2   'Spray and stretch' and other chilling methods – *cont'd*

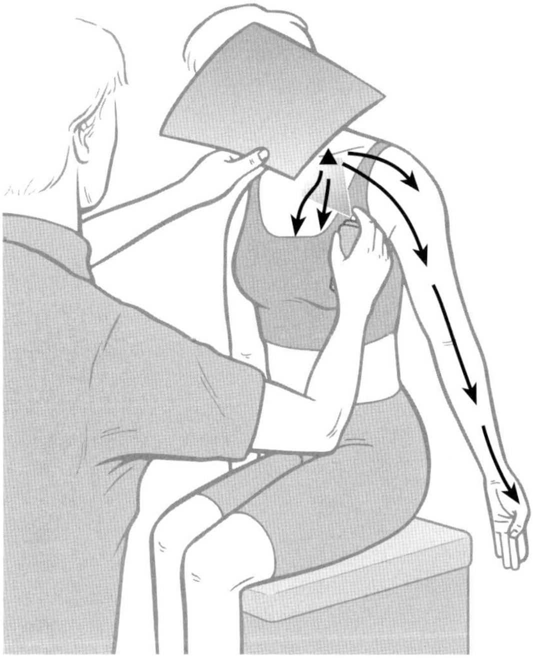

Figure 7.7   Use of spray ice to chill area between scalene muscle trigger point and the target area in the arm. Note that the head is side bent right and extended to stretch the left scalenes at the same time as the chilling takes place. (From Chaitow 2004.)

Box 7.3   Positional release technique (PRT)

Positional release methods were developed in osteopathic medicine. However, more recent evolutions of PRT – such as 'unloading taping' – have come from manual medicine and physical therapy sources.

At its simplest, positional release techniques involve placing tissues (muscles, joints, whole regions such as the low back or neck) into the most comfortable position possible.

This can be described as a 'position of ease', or 'comfort zone', or 'position of least resistance', and is identified by one of two methods:

1. Pain, which is being monitored by compression of a painful ('tender') point, reduces by at least 70% when the ease position is reached (when pain is used to guide tissues into ease, the method is called *strain/counterstrain*) (Jones 1981).
2. Tissues being palpated, but not pressed sufficiently to cause pain, are sensed to be at their most relaxed (when tissues are being palpated for their 'ease' position, with no pain being monitored, the method is called *functional technique*) (Bowles 1981, Greenman 1996, Hoover 1969).

There are a number of variations on these two themes (strain/counterstrain and functional technique), including amongst others orthobionomy, facilitated positional release and craniosacral technique.

All the variations, however, incorporate one or other of the two main protocols – ease the tissues, or ease the pain, and only strain/counterstrain (SCS) will be discussed in this chapter. For more information on PRT, three books are recommended:

1. Chaitow L 2003 *Positional Release Techniques*, 2nd edition. Churchill Livingstone, Edinburgh

Box 7.3   Positional release technique (PRT) – *cont'd*

2. D'Ambrogio K, Roth G 1997 *Positional Release Therapy.* Mosby, St Louis
3. Deig D 2001 *Positional Release Technique.* Butterworth-Heinemann, Boston.

SCS and trigger point – research evidence

Dardzinski et al (2000) evaluated the results of strain/counterstrain treatment combined with stretching techniques (self-applied by the patient) in individuals with myofascial/trigger point pain that had not responded to other forms of treatment.

Up to 75% of patients were significantly relieved of pain symptoms from the beginning of treatment, and this was largely maintained for 6 months, when patients were re-evaluated.

Main features of PRT

Both versions of PRT require that when tissues are being moved into an 'ease' position:

- all movements should be passive (therapist controls the movement, patient does nothing), and movements are slow and deliberate
- existing pain reduces, and no additional or new pain is created
- movement is away from restriction barriers
- muscle origins and insertions are brought together, rather than being stretched
- movement is away from any direction or position that causes pain or discomfort
- tissues being palpated soften
- painful tissues being palpated (possibly a trigger point) reduce in pain.

It is often the case that the position of ease is a replica of a position of strain that started whatever problem the patient now has.

This position of ease is reached in slow motion, painlessly and fully supported by the therapist.

Jones (1981) found that by taking the distressed joint (area) close to the position in which an original strain had taken place, muscle spindles that were protecting the area were given a chance to reset themselves, to become more relaxed, at which time pain in the area lessened.

The position of ease is also commonly an exaggeration of already distorted tissues. Again the tissues are taken into ease, slowly, painlessly and fully supported.

SCS guidelines

The general guidelines that Jones gives for relief of the dysfunction with which such tender points are related involves moving these tissues toward ease, which commonly involves the following elements.

- For tender points on the anterior surface of the body, flexion, side bending and rotation should be toward the palpated point, followed by fine-tuning to reduce sensitivity by at least 70% (Fig. 7.8).
- For tender points on the posterior surface of the body, extension, side bending and rotation should be away from the palpated point, followed by fine-tuning to reduce sensitivity by 70% (Fig. 7.9).
- The closer the tender point is to the midline, the less side bending and rotation should be required and the further from the midline, the more side bending and rotation should be required, in order to effect ease and comfort in the tender point (without any additional pain or discomfort being produced anywhere else).

The direction toward which side bending is introduced when trying to find a position of ease often needs to be away from the side of the palpated pain point, especially in relation to tender points found on the posterior aspect of the body.

The SCS process

- To use the strain/counterstrain (SCS) approach a painful point is located.
- This can be a 'tender' point, or an actual trigger point.
- Sufficient pressure is applied to the point to cause some pain.
- If it is a trigger point ensure that just enough pressure is being applied to cause the referred symptoms.
- The pain being felt is then given a value of 10.

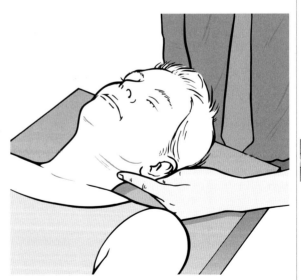

Figure 7.8   Treatment for C2–C6 side-flexion strain. (From Chaitow 2003a.)

Box 7.3   Positional release technique (PRT) – *cont'd*

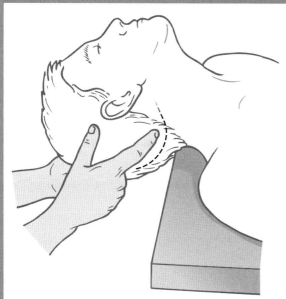

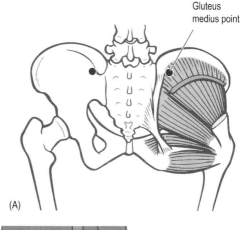

Gluteus medius point

(A)

Figure 7.9   First cervical extension strain. The position of ease requires extension of the neck and (usually) rotation away from the side of pain. (From Chaitow 2003a.)

- NOTE: This is not a situation in which the patient is asked to ascribe a pain level out of 10, instead it is one in which the question asked is 'Does the pressure hurt?'.
- If the answer is yes then the patient is told: 'Give the level of pain you are now feeling a value of 10, and as I move the area around and ask for feedback, give me the new pain level … whatever it is.'
- It is important to ask the patient to avoid comments such as 'It's increasing', or 'It's getting less', or any other verbal comment, other than a number.
- This helps to avoid undue delay in the process.
- In this example we can imagine that the tender, or trigger, point is in gluteus medius (Fig. 7.10).
- The patient would be prone, and the therapist would be applying sufficient pressure to the point to register pain which he/she would be told had a value of '10'.
- The supported leg on the side of pain would be moved in one direction (say extension at the hip) and the patient is asked what the pain is now.
- If the pain reduces another direction might be introduced (say adduction) … and the question is repeated.
- If the pain increased a different movement direction would be chosen.
- By gradually working through all the movement possibilities, in various directions, and possibly adding

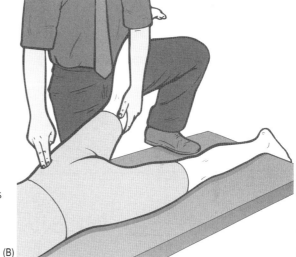

(B)

Figure 7.10   A: Gluteus medius tender point. B: Treatment of gluteus medius tender point. (From Chaitow 2003a.)

compression and distraction, a position would be found where pain drops by at least 70% (i.e. the score reaches 3 or less).
- Once this 'position of ease' has been found, after all the careful slow-motion fine-tuning, it would be maintained for not less than 90 seconds – and sometimes more – after which a slow return is made to the starting position.
- Range of motion, and degree of previous pain, should have changed for the better.
- In different tissues the possible directions of movement might include flexion, extension, rotation one way or the other, side flexion one way or the other, translation (shunting, or evaluating joint play)

Box 7.3   Positional release technique (PRT) – *cont'd*

as well as compression or distraction – to find the position of maximum ease.

The functional approach to finding 'ease'

In the functional approach, pain is not used as a guide to ease, but relaxation of tissues is palpated instead.

This achieves a similar position of ease to that found using the SCS method, but this time ease is found based on the palpation skill of the therapist, when the tissues are felt to be as soft and relaxed as possible.

Figure 7.11 shows a seated patient whose mid-back tissues are being palpated while the patient is slowly and carefully taken through all the variations of movement possible (arrows), until a combined position of maximum ease is achieved.

The patient is then held in this stress-free state for 90 seconds.

After that there would be a slow return to neutral; what was previously restricted will usually have a marked increase in range of motion, and will usually be very much less painful.

Unloading taping

In modern physical therapy methodology, particularly in athletic settings, joints and irritated tissues are taped into 'unloaded' positions, for hours and sometimes for days, while they recover from whatever has distressed them. This is a form of long-term positional release (Fig. 7.12).

What's happening when tissues are at ease?

What happens when tissues are at ease (whether 90 seconds or much longer)?

1. Pain receptors (nociceptors) reduce in sensitivity – something that is of importance where pain is a feature, whether this involves trigger points or not (Bailey & Dick 1992, Van Buskirk 1990).
2. In the comfort/ease position there is a marked improvement in blood flow and oxygenation through the tissues (Jacobson 1989). We know from the work of Travell & Simons (1983) that stressed soft tissues often contain localized areas of relative ischemia, lack of oxygen, and that this can be a key factor in

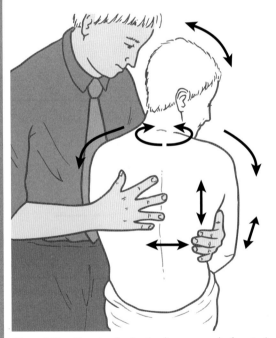

Figure 7.11   Functional palpation (or treatment) of a spinal region/segment during which all possible directions of motion are assessed for their influence on the sense of 'ease and bind' in the palpated tissues. After the first position of ease is identified (sequence is irrelevant) each subsequent assessment commences from the position of ease (or combined positions of ease) identified by the previous assessment(s) in a process known as 'stacking'. (From Chaitow 2003a.)

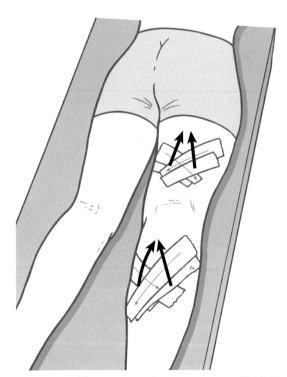

Figure 7.12   The tissues over the sciatic nerve are offloaded superiorly in the direction of the large arrows and the skin taped in the direction of the small arrows. (From Chaitow 2003a.)

Box 7.3   Positional release technique (PRT) – *cont'd*

production of pain and altered tissue status, which leads to the evolution of myofascial trigger points. Therefore improved oxygenation is of considerable importance, particularly to previously tense, ischemic muscles that are the natural breeding ground for trigger points.

3. Facilitated areas (spinal or trigger points) will be less active, less sensitized, calmer – less painful.

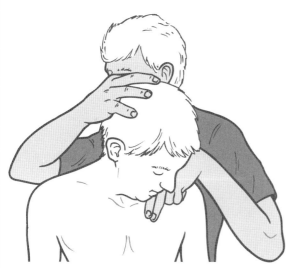

Figure 7.13   Pain and tissue tension is palpated and monitored. (From Chaitow 2003a.)

SCS as part of integrated neuromuscular inhibition technique

Strain/counterstrain is commonly used on its own when treating extremely acute and painful problems.

It is also used as part of a sequence of integrated methods that is used to treat trigger points, integrated neuromuscular inhibition technique (INIT). (This sequence is described fully in Box 7.6.)

Summary of PRT (Chaitow 2001, Jones 1981, Deig 2001)

- Locate and palpate a tender (or trigger) point if you are using SCS, or area of hypertonicity if using functional technique. See Figures 7.13 and 7.14 for examples of tender/trigger points being treated in the intercostal muscles and subclavius muscle.
- Tender (and trigger) points are most likely to be found in tense, shortened structures rather than relaxed ones.
- Use minimal force.
- Use minimal monitoring pressure.
- Achieve maximum ease/comfort/relaxation of tissues by slow movements of fine-tuning.
- Produce no additional pain anywhere else.
- Hold for 90 seconds.
- Return to neutral slowly.
- Retest range of motion and sensitivity.

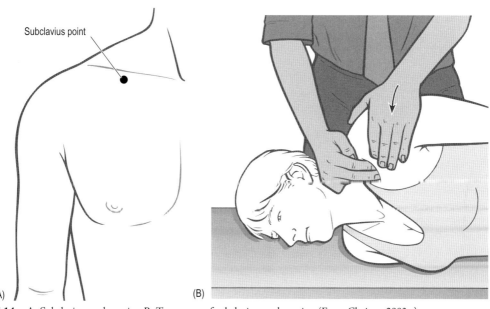

(A)   Subclavius point

(B)

Figure 7.14   A: Subclavius tender point. B: Treatment of subclavius tender point. (From Chaitow 2003a.)

Box 7.4   Muscle energy technique (MET) and other stretching methods

Simons, Travell & Simons (1999), the leading researchers into myofascial pain and the trigger point phenomenon, have made it absolutely clear: the muscle housing a trigger point must be restored to its normal resting length if reactivation of the trigger point activity is to be prevented.

Stretching therefore becomes a central part of the deactivation process.

This might involve:

1. stretching as a treatment on its own
2. stretching after compression (see Box 7.1)
3. stretching while the muscle is being chilled (see Box 7.2)
4. stretching as part of an integrated sequence that includes compression and positional release (INIT, see Box 7.6)
5. stretching after acupuncture or other needling methods have been used (see Box 9.1).

There are numerous ways of stretching.

The particular approach described in this chapter will be based on osteopathic muscle energy technique (MET) (Chaitow 2001).

This has similarities to PNF (proprioceptive neuromuscular facilitation) and a host of other variations such as active isolated stretching (Mattes 1995), hold-relax and contract-relax-antagonist-contract (CRAC), and facilitated stretching (McAtee & Charland 1999).

There is no suggestion that one method is superior to another, only that MET is the form of stretching with which the author is most familiar, and is therefore describing in this chapter.

MET is safe, effective, easy to use, and easy to teach to patients for self-use.

Example of added benefit from stretching in trigger point treatment

Hanten and colleagues (2000) compared the results of a home program of ischemic pressure and stretching, to a program of stretching alone, in people with trigger points in the trapezius muscle.

Ischemic pressure – combined with stretching – gave the most improvement in pain scores and raised pain pressure thresholds the most (i.e. more pressure was needed to cause pain).

As outlined in Box 7.1, the compression was always applied before the stretching.

Muscle energy technique (MET) variations (Greenman 1996, Janda 1989, Lewit 1999, Liebenson 1989, 1990, Simons et al 1999)

Definition: Muscle energy techniques are soft tissue

methods where the patient, on request, actively uses her muscles, in a specific direction, with mild effort, against a precise counterforce offered by the therapist (or gravity, or a fixed object such as a wall).

- If the counterforce matches the patient's effort this creates an isometric contraction. There is no movement with an *isometric contraction*; the forces are equal. This would happen, for example, if you pushed against an immovable object such as a wall. Another example is given in Figure 7.15, where the person is pushing her left elbow laterally while pushing against her elbow with her right hand to produce equal amounts of force (isometric). This would result in greater ease for stretching left side supraspinatus after the contraction.
- If the counterforce fails to match the patient's effort this is a *concentric isotonic contraction*. In Figure 7.16 the arm that is lifting the glass is overcoming resistance from the weight of the glass, the weight of the arm, and gravity. This is a concentric isotonic contraction.
- If the counterforce overcomes the patient's effort this is an *eccentric isotonic contraction*. In Figure 7.17 the flexor muscles of the arm that is putting the glass down are contracting as they lengthen so that the action is smooth and controlled, This is an eccentric isotonic contraction.

Two forms of MET

- If the muscle to be stretched is contracted isometrically the mechanism that allows easier stretching afterwards is called *post-isometric relaxation* (PIR) (Fig. 7.18).

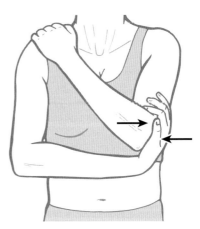

Figure 7.15   Position for stretching muscles between the shoulder blades on the left. (From Chaitow 2004.)

Box 7.4   Muscle energy technique (MET) and other stretching methods – *cont'd*

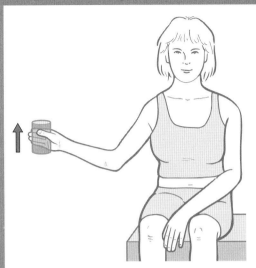

Figure 7.16   Lifting a glass of water is achieved by a concentric contraction. (From Chaitow 2004.)

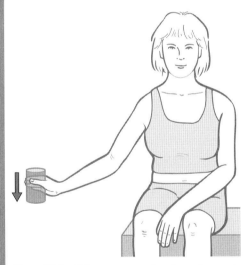

Figure 7.17   When you put a glass down the muscles are contracting while they are lengthening. This is an eccentric contraction. (From Chaitow 2004.)

- If the antagonist to the muscle to be stretched is contracted, the mechanism is called *reciprocal inhibition* (RI), which allows the tight muscle to be stretched more easily than it would without the contraction (Fig. 7.19).

Recent research (Ballantyne et al 2003) suggests that these two mechanisms, PIR and RI, are only part of the reason that stretching is easier after contractions of this sort. Although the precise mechanisms involved are not

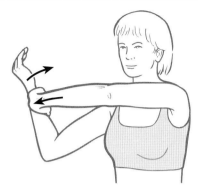

Figure 7.18   Contracting the shortened muscles against resistance so that no movement occurs (isometric contraction of the agonists) produces post-isometric relaxation (PIR). (From Chaitow 2004.)

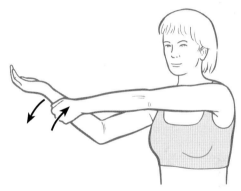

Figure 7.19   When the flexor muscles are tight, trying to straighten the arm against resistance without movement taking place at all (an isometric contraction of the antagonists) relaxes the flexor muscles by reciprocal inhibition. (From Chaitow 2004.)

yet clear (and RI and PIR are part of this), the process is simply labeled as '*increased stretch tolerance*'.

What this means is that after an isometric contraction the patient can tolerate more force being used to stretch soft tissues, with less discomfort than before the contraction.

Barrier rules and examples
To apply MET safely and effectively there are several basic 'rules' that need to applied:

- The 'barrier' from which the contraction is started refers to the very first sign of resistance to free movement, as the muscle is taken toward its end of range. The feeling that the barrier has been reached is described as a sense of tension, or 'bind'.

Box 7.4 Muscle energy technique (MET) and other stretching methods – cont'd

- It is from this barrier that MET should be started.

Take, for example, a tight hamstring group of muscles (Fig. 7.20).

- The patient's left side hamstring group has been taken to its first resistance barrier.
- For about 5 to 7 seconds the patient, on instruction from the therapist, contracts the hamstrings by attempting to take the leg back to the table, using about 20% of his strength, fully resisted by the therapist.
- After the isometric contraction (as defined above), because of PIR, the leg will be easier to move beyond the previous barrier, into stretch.
- This stretch would be held for about 30 seconds, to introduce a lengthening (stretching) effect.
- The process should then be repeated.
- None of these elements should produce any pain.

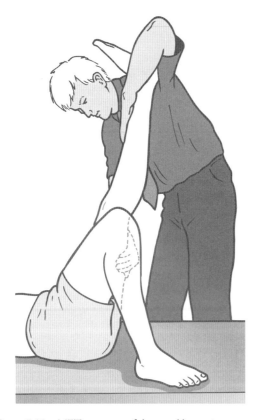

Figure 7.20 MET treatment of shortened hamstrings. Following an isometric contraction, the leg is taken to or through the resistance barrier (depending on whether the problem is acute or chronic). (From Chaitow 2001.)

- If the contraction itself is painful then the alternative method (RI) should be used.
- This time, instead of contracting the hamstrings (by trying to take the leg back to the table against resistance), the patient would contract the quadriceps, by being asked to raise the leg further, against resistance (provided by the therapist), for 7 seconds, using no more than 20% of strength.
- This would produce RI and would allow a stretch of the hamstrings to be more easily introduced.
- If the stretch itself is painful then the muscle is being taken too far past its barrier of resistance.

Use of eye movement (Simons et al 1999)

Eye movements are sometimes used during contractions and stretches. This is because an automatic increase in muscle tone occurs in muscles, as they prepare to move in the direction in which the eyes are looking.

This visual synkinesis (to give its full name) is useful when muscles are too painful to contract, and is particularly useful in the neck and shoulder region.

Try a small experiment.

- Sit with the head facing forward.
- Move your eyes only to look as far to the left as you can and while holding the eyes in this position turn your head to the right.
- When you have turned your head as far right as you can, while still looking left, shift your eyes to look right, and you should now be able to take your head much further to the right.

This shows how much extra tone is created by the eye movement alone.

To use this in treatment have the patient look in a direction that will tone particular muscles.

For example, you could ask the supine patient to 'look down your nose toward your feet for a few seconds', to introduce a mild contraction of the anterior neck muscles, such as scalene and sternomastoid.

After 5 to 7 seconds you could ask the patient to close the eyes, as you gently stretch these muscles.

Main MET applications

MET is ideal for:

- relaxing acute muscular spasm or contraction (using PIR or RI as discussed above)
- mobilizing restricted joints (using PIR or RI as discussed above)
- preparing muscles for stretching (using PIR or RI as discussed above)
- MET is also used as part of the INIT trigger point deactivation sequence (see Box 7.6).

Box 7.4   Muscle energy technique (MET) and other stretching methods – *cont'd*

In addition:

- isotonic concentric contractions are used for toning muscles or rehabilitation
- isotonic eccentric contractions are used to tone the antagonists of tight muscles, and to prepare these for stretching
- there are also variations such as isokinetic and 'pulsed' MET methods that have specialized use.

MET for local stretching

When MET is used as part of the INIT sequence for trigger point deactivation (see Box 7.6), it is involved in two parts of that process:

1. a local area of muscle, directly around the trigger point, should be isometrically contracted and then stretched, after which,
2. the whole muscle should be isometrically contracted and then stretched.

In order to achieve the local stretch a very focused isometric contraction is needed, and this is achieved as follows:

- Using ischemic compression on the trigger.
- Easing the pain from that compression by at least 70% by positioning (as described in Box 7.3).
- While holding the tissues in their 'ease' position (folded around the trigger point usually), a local isometric contraction, involving those very 'folded' tissues, is asked for (see Box 7.6 for more detail).
- The local tissues housing the trigger point are then put at stretch.
- Figure 7.21 shows a local stretch applied to part of the rectus abdominis muscle. In this example, the trigger would lie between the two thumbs.
- Figure 7.22 shows a local stretch of part of the iliotibial band. Again the trigger lies between the two thumbs.
- The whole muscle is then contracted isometrically.
- The whole muscle is then stretched.
- In the description of stretching of tissues relating to scar tissue, in Box 7.5, there are indications as to how to introduce local stretching.

Examples of whole muscle stretches using MET

In Chapter 4 there are maps showing most of the areas that can be affected by trigger points, with indications of which muscles might be involved in relation to each area.

A selection of MET whole muscle stretches are illustrated below to assist in visualizing just how that element of trigger point deactivation might be achieved.

For full descriptions and video clips (on CD ROM) see *Muscle Energy Techniques*, 2nd edition (Chaitow 2001).

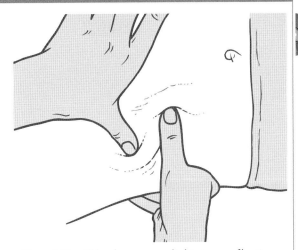

Figure 7.21   'S' bend pressure applied to tense or fibrotic musculature. (From Chaitow 2003b.)

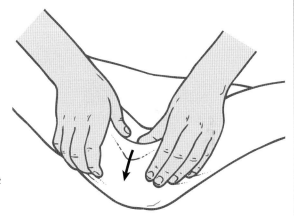

Figure 7.22   'C' bend pressure. (From Chaitow 2003b)

NOTE: The examples of particular muscles illustrated below are by no means all the possible variations that can be treated by MET, but are meant as illustrations of:

- suggested MET positions for initiating stretch into the muscles illustrated
- the pain distribution of active trigger points in those muscles.

For more widespread trigger point influences see the maps in Chapter 4 – including the illustrations of referral patterns into the face and head of trigger points in that region (Figs 4.10 to 4.15).

Also review Figure 2.11 in Chapter 2, which illustrates a variety of trigger point locations and referral zones.

Box 7.4   Muscle energy technique (MET) and other stretching methods – *cont'd*

Rectus femoris (Fig. 7.23)
Trigger points in this muscle may refer pain to:

- lateral thigh and hip
- anterior thigh
- anterior knee
- anteromedial knee.

Lower hamstrings (Fig. 7.24)
Trigger points in this muscle may refer pain to:

- buttocks
- posterior thigh
- posterior leg
- posterior knee.

Tensor fascia lata (Fig. 7.25)
Trigger points in this muscle may refer pain to:

- lateral thigh and hip.

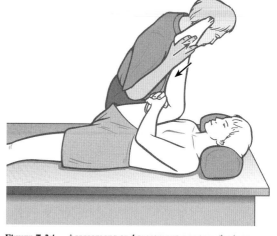

Figure 7.24   Assessment and treatment position for lower hamstring fibers. (From Chaitow 2001.)

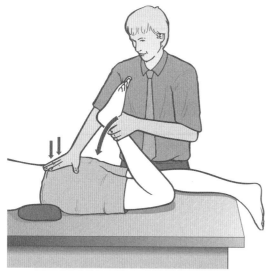

Figure 7.23   MET treatment of left rectus femoris muscle. Note the practitioner's right hand stabilizes the sacrum and pelvis to prevent undue stress during the stretching phase of the treatment. (From Chaitow 2001.)

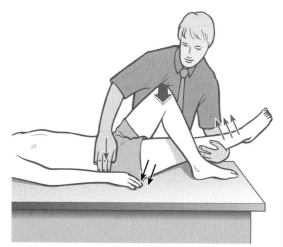

Figure 7.25   MET treatment of tensor fascia lata. If a standard MET method is being used, the stretch will follow the isometric contraction in which the patient will attempt to move the right leg to the right against sustained resistance. It is important for the practitioner to maintain stability of the pelvis during the procedure. (From Chaitow 2001.)

Box 7.4   Muscle energy technique (MET) and other stretching methods – *cont'd*

Piriformis (Figs 7.26 and 7.27)
Trigger points in this muscle may refer pain to:

- buttocks
- lateral thigh and hip
- posterior thigh
- pelvis
- sacrum and gluteal area.

Quadratus lumborum (Fig. 7.28)
Trigger points in this muscle may refer pain to:

- sacrum and gluteal area
- abdomen
- buttock
- sacroiliac joint
- lateral thigh.

Upper trapezius (Fig. 7.29)
Trigger points in this muscle may refer pain to:

- neck and head
- upper thoracic area
- back of shoulder
- mid-thoracic spine.

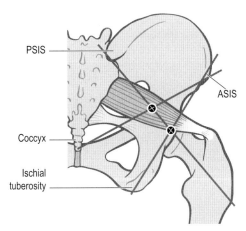

Figure 7.26   Using bony landmarks as coordinates, the commonest tender areas are located in piriformis, in the belly and at the attachment of the muscle. PSIS, posterior superior iliac spine; ASIS, anterior superior iliac spine. (From Chaitow 2001.)

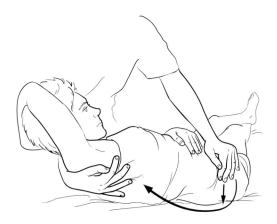

Figure 7.28   MET treatment of quadratus lumborum utilizing 'banana' position. (From Chaitow 2001.)

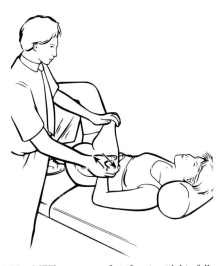

Figure 7.27   MET treatment of piriformis with hip fully flexed and externally rotated. (From Chaitow 2001.)

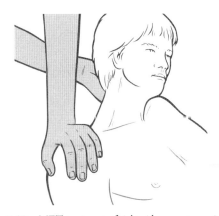

Figure 7.29   MET treatment of right side upper trapezius muscle – middle fibers. (From Chaitow 2001.)

Box 7.4   Muscle energy technique (MET) and other stretching methods – *cont'd*

Scalenes (Fig. 7.30)

Trigger points in this muscle may refer pain to:

- back of shoulder
- upper thoracic area
- front of chest ('pseudo angina')
- mid-thoracic area
- back of arm (scalenus minimus)
- front of arm (scalenus minimus)
- radial forearm
- dorsal finger area
- base of thumb and radial hand area.

Levator scapulae (Fig. 7.31)

Trigger points in this muscle may refer pain to:

- upper thoracic area
- back of shoulder
- mid-thoracic area.

Pectoralis major (Fig. 7.32)

Trigger points in this muscle may refer pain to:

- front of shoulder
- medial epicondyle
- ulnar forearm
- wrist and palm
- dorsal aspects of fingers
- front of chest.

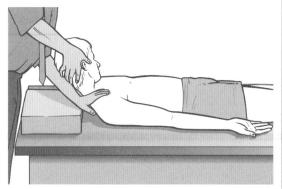

Figure 7.31   MET test and treatment position for levator scapula (right side). (From Chaitow 2001.)

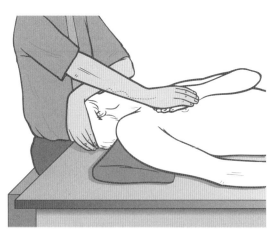

Figure 7.30   MET treatment for the middle fibers of scalenes. The hand placement (thenar of hypothenar eminence of relaxed hand) is on the second rib below the center of the clavicle. (From Chaitow 2001.)

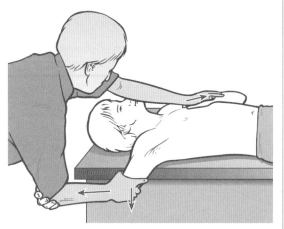

Figure 7.32   An alternative hold for application of MET to pectoral muscle – sternal attachment. Note that the patient needs to be close to the edge of the table in order to allow the arm to be taken towards the floor once the slack has been removed, during the stretching phase after the isometric contraction. (From Chaitow 2001.)

Box 7.5   Myofascial release (MFR) and skin release for scar tissue

Myofascial release is a soft tissue technique that helps the stretching of restricted fascia. Sustained, steady but not excessive, pressure is applied against tissue barriers, and after 90 to 120 seconds the tissue lengthens, allowing a release to be felt.

The therapist then follows the release holding pressure against the new tissue barrier and holds.

After several such releases the tissues will become softer and more pliable (Barnes 1996, Shea 1993).

The dense 'gel' state of connective tissue yields to sustained moderate pressure by becoming increasingly 'sol' (solute), softer and more pliable.

Fascial tissues lengthen in response to pressure – a process known as 'creep' (Twomey & Taylor 1982).

As the tissues change in length (deform) there is a heat and energy exchange, known as hysteresis (*Dorland's* 1985).

A number of different techniques are used to achieve MFR:

- Pressure is applied to restricted myofascia using a 'curved' contact and direction of pressure in an attempt to glide or slide against the restriction barrier.
- The patient may be asked to assist by means of breathing tactics or by moving the area in a way that enhances the release, based on practitioner instructions.
- As softening occurs, the direction of pressure is reassessed and gradually applied to move toward a new restriction barrier.

Mock (1997) describes a different, progressive, model of MFR that includes stages or 'levels':

1. Level 1 involves treatment of tissues without introducing tension. The practitioner's contact (which could involve hand, thumb, finger, knuckle or elbow) moves along the muscle fibers, distal to proximal, with the patient passive, a form of effleurage.
2. Level 2 is precisely the same, but in this instance the glide/effleurage strokes are applied to muscle which has been placed in tension (at slight stretch).
3. Level 3 involves the introduction of passively induced motion, as an area of restriction is compressed while the tissues are taken passively through their fullest possible range of motion, a rhythmic stretching and wringing of the tissues.
4. Level 4 is the same but this time the patient actively moves the tissues through the fullest possible range of motion, from shortest to longest, while the therapist offers resistance.

These two models of myofascial release, the first taking tissue to the elastic barrier and waiting for a release mechanism to operate, and the second involving force being applied to induce change.

Whichever approach is adopted, MFR technique is used to improve movement potentials, reduce restrictions, release spasm, ease pain and restore normal function to previously dysfunctional tissues, commonly housing trigger points.

A similarity can be seen with MET methods, because the fundamental effect is to lengthen shortened soft tissues, and in the process to improve circulation and oxygenation. Lewit (1999) has described the process as 'shifting' the fascial tissue rather than 'stretching' it.

Whatever we describe it as, shifting or stretching, these effects of MFR will automatically inhibit and commonly deactivate trigger points.

Example: paraspinal myofascial release

To treat tense, shortened soft tissues that house trigger points in the paraspinal lumbar muscles:

- You stand to the side of the prone patient, facing the patient at waist level contralateral to the side to be treated.
- Cross your arms so that a separation force can easily be introduced.
- Your cephalad hand is placed on the paraspinal region close to the crest of the pelvis, facing caudad.
- Your caudad hand is placed, fingers facing cephalad, on the lower thorax, so that the heels of the hands are a few centimeters apart and on the same side of the torso.
- If a trigger point is being targeted it should lie in tissues deep to your contact hands, between them.
- Light compression is applied into the tissues, one hand taking out slack in a cephalad and the other in a caudad direction, until each hand reaches the elastic barrier of the tissues being contacted.
- Pressure is *not* applied into the torso – instead, traction (separation) occurs on the superficial tissues, which lie between the two hands.
- These barriers are held for not less than 90 seconds, and commonly between 2 and 3 minutes, until a sense of separation of the tissues is noted.
- The tissues are followed to their new barriers, and the light, sustained separation force is maintained until a further release is sensed.
- The superficial fascia will have been released, and the status of associated myofascial tissues will be improved (Fig. 7.33).

Box 7.5   Myofascial release (MFR) and skin release for scar tissue – *cont'd*

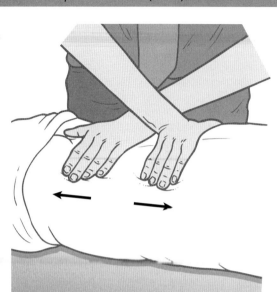

Figure 7.33   Cross-handed myofascial release. (From Barnes 1997.)

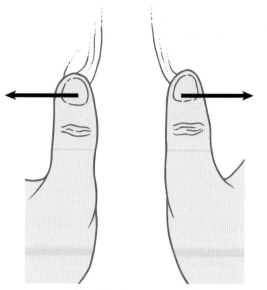

Figure 7.34   Holding skin (close to scar tissue) at stretch to begin process of trigger point deactivation.

Scar tissue myofascial release methods

The skin assessment methods detailed in Chapter 6 (drag, loss of elasticity, etc.) allow skin alongside scars to be easily assessed for change.

If such skin is tight/tense, and/or displays a sense of drag as you run a finger lightly over it, it is important to see whether it produces symptoms when lightly stretched, or pressed.

Using two fingers you hold the skin at its barrier of stretch for around 10 seconds (Fig. 7.34).

This is a mini-myofascial release.

Alternatively 'S' and 'C' bends can be introduced, taking the tissues (skin and underlying fascia) to their elastic barrier until a release occurs (Fig. 7.35).

Instead of two hands you have two fingers, or two thumbs, performing the engagement of the resistance barrier, waiting for release.

After 10 to 15 seconds (sometimes far less), tension should be felt to weaken so that a normal springiness is restored to the skin.

Retesting for drag or 'tightness' should now show normal, rather than abnormal, skin responses (Lewit 1999).

In German the word *Störungsfeld* – 'focus of disturbance' – is used.

This describes an old scar, the result of injury or surgery, tender on examination, with pain spots (sometimes referring like trigger points) and altered skin function surrounding it.

The skin displays drag characteristics, and/or tightness in the skin when taken to its elastic barrier.

Lewit has found that these areas need special attention.

He suggests deep palpation for painful (often trigger) points, near scars.

If there is a feeling of tissue resistance ('adhesions') and/or drag, or loss of skin elasticity (as described in Chapter 6), then treatment should start with skin stretching as described above.

If release of the skin by stretching fails to normalize the pain point, and the skin status, then needling might be called for.

Lewit suggests that more often than not skin stretching and/or 'springing' is all that is needed.

Box 7.5   Myofascial release (MFR) and skin release for scar tissue – *cont'd*

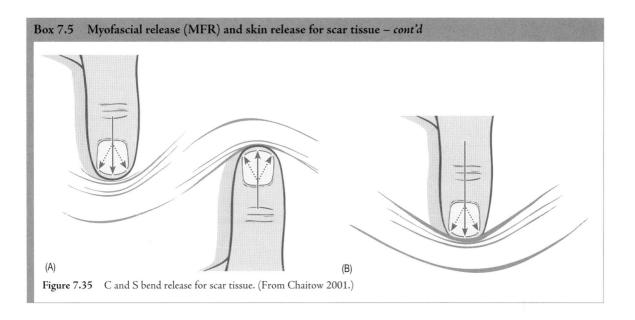

(A)   (B)

Figure 7.35   C and S bend release for scar tissue. (From Chaitow 2001.)

Box 7.6   INIT: Integrated neuromuscular inhibition technique (Chaitow 1994)

INIT method

An integrated treatment sequence has been developed for the deactivation of myofascial trigger points. The method is as follows:

1. The trigger point is identified by palpation.
2. Ischemic compression is applied in either a sustained or intermittent manner (see Box 7.1 for variations in how to apply compression).
3. When referred or local pain starts to reduce in intensity, the compression treatment stops.
4. The patient should be told something such as: *'I am going to press that same point again, and I want you to give the pain that you feel a "value" of 10. I will then gently reposition the area and you will feel differences in the levels of pain. In some positions the pain may increase, in others it will decrease. When I ask you for feedback as to what's happening to the pain, please give me a number out of 10. If the pain has increased it may go up – to say 11 or 12. Just give me the number you are feeling. We are aiming to find a position in which the pain drops to 3 or less, and the more accurately you give me the "pain score" the faster I will be able to fine-tune the process, so that we can get to the "comfort" position.'*
5. Using the methods outlined in Box 7.3, the tissues housing the trigger point are then carefully placed in a position of ease with the patient's help.
6. This ease position is held for approximately 20–30 seconds, to allow neurological resetting, reduction in

pain receptor activity, and enhanced local circulation/oxygenation.

7. An isometric contraction is then focused into the musculature around the trigger point to create post-isometric relaxation (PIR) (see Box 7.5).
8. The way this is done varies with the particular part of the body being treated. Sometimes all that is necessary is to say to the patient, *'Tighten the muscles around the place where my thumb is pressing'.* At other times, if the patient is being supported in a position of ease, it may be helpful to say something such as: *'I am going to let go of your leg* (or neck, or arm, or whatever else you are supporting) *and I want you to hold the position on your own for a few seconds'.* In one way or another you need to induce a contraction of the muscle tissues around the trigger point so that they can be stretched.
9. After the contraction (5 to 7 seconds, with the patient using only a small amount of effort) the soft tissues housing the trigger point are stretched locally (see Fig 7.35, and also Figs 7.21 and 7.22).
10. The local stretch is important because it is often the case in a large muscle (such as the hamstrings) that stretching the whole muscle will effectively lengthen it, but the tight bundle where the trigger point is situated will be relatively unstretched – like a knot in a piece of elastic which remains knotted even though the elastic is held at stretch.
11. After holding the local stretch (see Figs 7.23 to 7.32 and also 7.33) for approximately 30 seconds the

Box 7.6   INIT: Integrated neuromuscular inhibition technique (Chaitow 1994) – *cont'd*

entire muscle should then be contracted and stretched – again holding that stretch for at least 30 seconds (Figs 7.36 and 7.37).

12. The patient should assist in stretching movements (whenever possible) by activating the antagonists and so facilitating the stretch.

13. A towel that has been rung out in warm/hot water placed over the treated tissues for 5 to 10 minutes helps to ease the soreness that may follow this treatment.

14. Within 24 hours the trigger should have reduced in activity considerably, or no longer be active. Retesting immediately after the INIT sequence may not offer evidence of this, as tissues will be tender.

INIT rationale

When a trigger point is being palpated by direct finger or thumb pressure, and when the very tissues in which the trigger point lies are positioned in such a way as to take away the pain (entirely or at least by 70%), the most

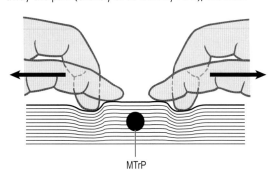

MTrP

Figure 7.36   This local stretch is designed to precisely lengthen the shortened fibers of a myofascial trigger point following a localized, focused isometric contraction.

(dis)stressed fibers, in which trigger points are housed, are in a position of relative ease (see Box 7.3).

The trigger point is under direct inhibitory pressure (mild or perhaps intermittent – see Box 7.1) while positioned so that the tissues housing it are relaxed (relatively or completely).

Following a period of 20–30 seconds of this position of ease, the patient is asked to introduce a mild (20% of strength) isometric contraction into the tissues (against the practitioner's resistance) and to hold this for 5 to 7 seconds, involving the very fibers involved in the positional release positioning.

After the contraction, a reduction in tone will have been induced in the tissues (PIR) – see Box 7.4.

The hypertonic or fibrotic tissues can then be stretched more easily than they could before the contraction (as in any muscle energy procedure) so that the specifically targeted fibers are lengthened.

Wherever possible, the patient assists in this stretching movement in order to activate the antagonists and facilitate the stretch.

The advantage of this combination is that it is open to variation. For example, in very sensitive individuals the sustained compression element can be reduced and the trigger point taken immediately into its ease position, followed by stretching.

Research by Hou et al (2002) and Hong (1994) shows that combinations of methods are more successful in deactivating trigger points than single methods used alone (e.g. only stretching, or only compression).

The protocol outlined above (INIT) offers a flexible combination of methods, all of which have been shown to be successful when used on their own.

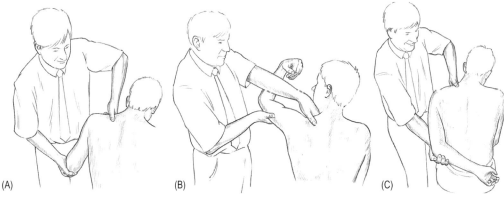

(A)   (B)   (C)

Figure 7.37   A: First stage of INIT in which a tender/pain/trigger point in supraspinatus is located and ischemically compressed, either intermittently or persistently. B: The pain is removed from the tender/pain/trigger point by finding a position of ease which is held for at least 20 seconds, following which an isometric contraction is achieved involving the tissues that house the tender/pain/trigger point. C: Following the holding of the isometric contraction for an appropriate period, the muscle housing the point of local soft tissue dysfunction is stretched. This completes the INIT sequence. (From Chaitow 2001.)

Box 7.7   Manipulation, mobilization

In her very early writings Janet Travell (1942), the main pioneer of trigger point research, suggested that high-velocity low-amplitude thrust – HVLT – (as used in chiropractic and some osteopathic manipulation) was a useful part of patient care. And the most recent revision of her main text (collaborating with David and Lois Simons) continues to suggest the value of manipulation when dealing with myofascial pain (Simons et al 1999).

Is there evidence to support the use of HVLT in treating trigger point dysfunction?

De las Peñas (2004) has reviewed all recent research that looks at manual methods of trigger point treatment.

Amongst these are studies that report on the use of mobilization and manipulation, such as occipital release and active head retraction and retraction/extension movements in treatment of cervical and scapula trigger points (Hanten et al 1997).

De las Peñas (2004) reports that, because these mobilization methods were frequently used in combination with massage and/or compression, and because both compression and massage have been shown to have beneficial effects on myofascial pain (see Boxes 7.1 and 7.9), there is no evidence that mobilization and manipulation offer any additional benefit.

Various chiropractic researchers have compared manipulation (high-velocity low-amplitude thrust/HVLT) used on its own with other forms of manual treatment ('physical modalities') in combination with chiropractic (HVLT) manipulation (Haas et al 2004, Hurwitz et al 2002).

These modalities included massage (in 75% of the patients), and use of ice treatment (see Box 7.2) in over 90% of the patients. Some patients also received 'trigger point' treatment (unspecified as to what this comprised) as well.

Results showed that the chronic low back pain of patients receiving both forms of treatment (HVLT or HVLT together with other physical modalities) improved, with significant reduction in 'spot tenderness' in spinal regions.

Those receiving the combination treatment (massage, compression, etc.) improved more than those receiving only manipulation.

The conclusion must be that when it is indicated, manipulation probably assists in normalization of dysfunction, but that soft tissue treatment (i.e. massage, compression, stretching, plus use of ice) probably helps more, especially when these methods are used in combination and not alone.

Box 7.8   Manual lymphatic drainage

Lymphatic drainage techniques
Lymphatic drainage is designed to improve lymphatic flow.

The nature of manual lymphatic drainage (MLD) demands that the therapist has very good knowledge of the anatomy of the lymphatic system, as well as being well trained in the extreme delicacy required to achieve increased flow/drainage, without traumatizing the delicate structures involved (Figs 7.38 and 7.39).

Pressure used in lymph drainage should be very light indeed, less than an ounce (28 g) per cm^2 (under 8 oz per square inch), in order to encourage lymph flow, without increasing blood filtration.

This level of pressure would be what is tolerable to your eyeballs, if you applied pressure to them with your fingers.

According to Harris & Piller (2004) the maximum amount of pressure used in MLD should not be greater than 32 mmHg. This can be experienced by placing a blood pressure (sphygmomanometer) cuff around your arm, and inflating this to 32 mmHg.

You will feel that the pressure is very, very light indeed.

MLD characteristics
Harris & Piller (2004) summarize the characteristics of MLD when applying one of the five basic techniques (stationary circles, thumb circles, pump technique, scoop technique, rotary technique):

1. light rhythmic alternating pressure with each stroke
2. skin stretching and torque both lengthwise and diagonally
3. pressure and stretch applied in direction of desired fluid flow (not always in direction of lymph flow)
4. light pressure over spongy edematous areas and slightly firmer over fibrotic tissue
5. pressure not to exceed 32 mmHg.

When to use MLD
It is suggested that practitioners/therapists trained in lymphatic drainage should apply lymphatic drainage techniques before neuromuscular or other deep tissue procedures, in order to prepare the tissues for treatment, as well as after NMT/deep tissue procedures to remove excessive waste products from the tissues (Chaitow & DeLany 2000).

Box 7.8　Manual lymphatic drainage – *cont'd*

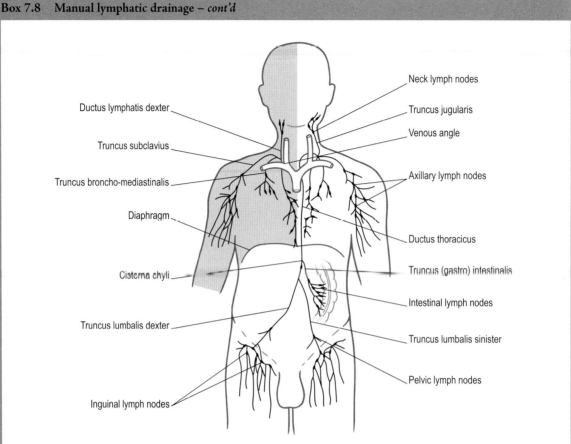

Neck lymph nodes

Truncus jugularis

Venous angle

Axillary lymph nodes

Ductus thoracicus

Truncus (gastro) intestinalis

Intestinal lymph nodes

Truncus lumbalis sinister

Pelvic lymph nodes

Ductus lymphatis dexter

Truncus subclavius

Truncus broncho-mediastinalis

Diaphragm

Cisterna chyli

Truncus lumbalis dexter

Inguinal lymph nodes

Figure 7.38　Major lymph trunks in the body, and their drainage areas. (Reproduced with permission, from Foldi & Strossenreuther 2005.)

MLD and trigger points

It is claimed that individual trigger points can be deactivated using MLD methods alone; however, there is no research validation of this claim, only a substantial amount of anecdotal evidence (Chikly 1997, 1999).

Trigger points and lymphatic flow problems

Trigger point activity has been shown by Simons et al (1999) to interfere with lymphatic flow in a number of ways:

- Scalene trigger points (especially in anterior scalene) cause tension that interferes with drainage into the thoracic duct.

- This is aggravated by first rib restrictions that can result from trigger points in middle and posterior scalenes.
- The movement of lymph by means of peristaltic contractions is interfered with by scalene trigger points.
- Trigger points in subscapularis, teres major and latissimus dorsi, in the posterior axillary folds, slow down lymphatic flow, affecting the arms and breast tissues.
- Trigger points in the anterior axillary area (pectoralis minor in particular) influence lymphatic drainage of the breasts (Zink 1981).

Box 7.8   Manual lymphatic drainage – *cont'd*

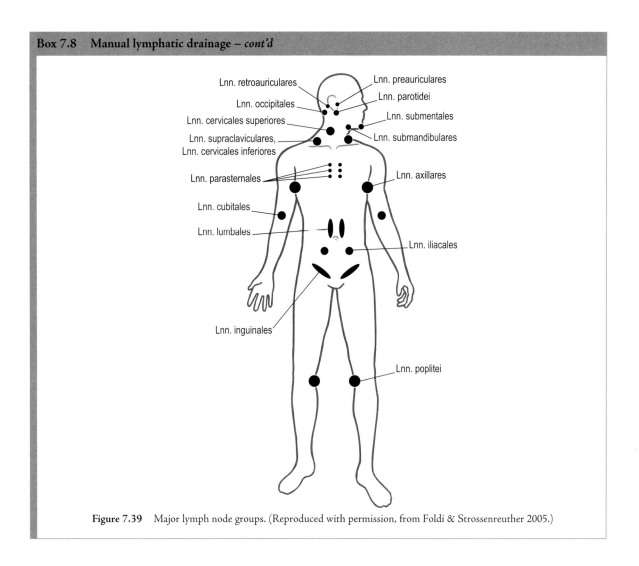

Lnn. retroauriculares
Lnn. preauriculares
Lnn. occipitales
Lnn. parotidei
Lnn. cervicales superiores
Lnn. submentales
Lnn. supraclaviculares,
Lnn. submandibulares
Lnn. cervicales inferiores
Lnn. parasternales
Lnn. axillares
Lnn. cubitales
Lnn. lumbales
Lnn. iliacales
Lnn. inguinales
Lnn. poplitei

Figure 7.39   Major lymph node groups. (Reproduced with permission, from Foldi & Strossenreuther 2005.)

Box 7.9   Massage

It is not easy to define massage. Does it include compression methods? Does it include stretching techniques?

According to Fritz (1998), compression and stretching are basic techniques used in traditional massage, whether this is so-called 'wellness' massage, or Swedish, or therapeutic massage.

Certainly, when writing about compression methods, as well as about focused local stretching (as illustrated in Box 7.5), Simons (2002) describes all these methods as 'massage'.

This makes massage (in all its forms) an ideal trigger point treatment approach.

Recent research confirms the value of massage for treatment of trigger points responsible for symptoms such as pelvic pain and interstitial cystitis (Oyama et al 2004, Weiss 2001).

For example, one research study involved 42 people with chronic cystitis, whose main symptoms were painful urgency and frequency.

After manual treatment of myofascial trigger points located in the pelvic muscles (using compression and stretching method), 35 of these people (83%) reported moderate to marked improvement.

Some were completely relieved of their symptoms, after enduring them for up to 14 years. Seven of the 10 people who had been diagnosed with a condition known as *interstitial cystitis* showed moderate to marked improvements after trigger point deactivation (Weiss 2001).

Swedish massage

A summary by Rachlin (1994) indicated that, although some types of superficial massage, such as those consisting of stroking and kneading, are good for general relaxation, simply massaging the area of reported pain, without trying to find and eradicate trigger points that may be responsible, will not provide the patient with lasting relief.

A combination of deep and superficial massage for treatment of trigger points was therefore suggested by Rachlin. The recommended techniques consist of an initial period of Swedish massage-like techniques, including stroking, kneading and stripping, to warm the tissue and make it more elastic, after which you will be more able to apply increased pressure, deep into the muscle, with reduced discomfort for the patient.

Similarly, when treating low back pain associated with trigger points, Preyde (2000) reported a reduction in pain after 4 weeks of comprehensive massage, involving soft tissue manipulation, consisting of deep friction, trigger point and neuromuscular therapy, combined with stretching exercises.

Thai massage

The effectiveness and benefits of traditional Thai massage (TTM) for patients with back pain associated with myofascial trigger points was compared with superficial Western (Swedish) massage (Chatchawan et al 2005).

In this study 180 patients with myofascial pain symptoms received either TTM or superficial Western (Swedish) massage (SM), twice weekly, for 3 weeks

TTM was performed according to the system of Royal Thai massage, which is based on the concept of invisible energy lines running through the body (similar to the meridians of traditional Chinese medicine).

(Note: European neuromuscular technique – NMT – was derived, in the 1930s, from traditional Ayurvedic (Indian) massage methods that had as an objective the release of superficial obstructions to the flow of energy – *prana*, the equivalent of the Chinese *chi*)

Massage points, included in TTM treatment, are located on two of these lines, lying on each side of the spine (Fig. 7.40).

The first line of massage starts from a point 2 cm (about an inch) above the posterior superior iliac spine (PSIS), and ends at the thoracocervical junction. Each point on this line is approximately 1 finger width to the side of each spinous process.

The second line follows the same course, but is about 2 finger widths to the side of each spinous process.

There are also two additional massage points, one on each side of the low back, located 3 finger widths away from the spinous process of the L2 vertebra (Fig. 7.40).

Method of TTM used in this study

- The TTM pressing technique uses the therapist's body weight to apply gentle, gradually increasing, pressure through the thumb, finger, palm and/or elbow.
- Pressure is applied until the patient starts to feel some pain (just past the pain threshold), after which the pressure is maintained for 5–10 seconds (Prateepavanich et al 1999).
- This sequence is repeated several times, on each massage point.

Superficial massage (SM)

- The SM treatment that was compared with TTM in this research was performed using jojoba oil.
- Pressure was applied on the area of the back between PSIS and C7.
- This pressure was sufficient to reach deep into the subcutaneous tissue, but was not sufficient to exceed the pain threshold.
- SM techniques were adapted from Swedish massage, and included superficial stroking, effleurage and

---

Box 7.9   Massage – *cont'd*

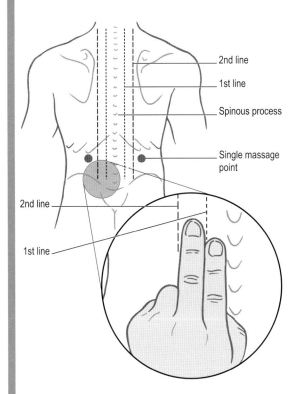

Figure 7.40   Points related to traditional Thai massage. (From Chatchawan et al 2005.)

petrissage – including kneading (with the thumb, fingers, and palm), wringing, and skin rolling.

Results
Results showed that both methods (TTM and SM) were equally effective in reducing trigger point pain symptoms by approximately 50%.

At follow-up, a month after treatment had stopped, the levels of pain relief had been maintained.

In other studies TTM has been shown to produce powerful pain-relieving effects, and to be an effective means for deactivating trigger points (Prateepavanich et al 1999).

Survey of massage and trigger points
The best research available into manual methods of trigger point treatment has been reviewed by de las Peñas (2004).

He lists studies by Gam et al (1998), Hanten et al (2000), Hong (1994), Hou et al (2002), and others, that included either 'soft tissue' massage, compression, myofascial release and spray and stretch, or combinations of these and other modalities (ultrasound, TENS, etc.).

For example, de las Peñas (2004) discusses Hanten et al (2000) who compared the results of a program of stretching alone, to a home program of ischemic pressure and stretching, in people with trigger points in the trapezius region.

Ischemic pressure, combined with stretching, produced a greater improvement in pain scores and pain pressure threshold, than stretching on its own.

Hanten et al's research shows the added benefit of different massage techniques (compression methods as described in Box 7.1) when used together.

Overall, the conclusion of the survey is the confirmation that treatment of trigger points is effective in reducing pressure pain sensitivity, and that improvements commonly occurred using different manual therapies in combination (spray and stretch, deep pressure, soft tissue massage and ischemic compression).

Massage (including compression and stretching methods) appears to be a key feature of the most effective manual methods.

Box 7.10   Education/rehabilitation and self-help

All healthcare professions work with a constant and unfailing ally.

This ally is the self-healing, self-regulating action of the body–mind complex.

We get better after most injuries. We recover from most illnesses. Broken bones mend. Cuts heal. Infections are overcome by our immune systems, and so on.

Or, more accurately, these statements are true, *if* the self-regulating systems and mechanisms of the body are working properly.

Cuts do not heal, infections are not overcome, and broken bones do not mend … if circumstances exist that prevent the normal processes from taking place.

We have seen a great deal of evidence for the fact that pain and dysfunction can frequently be caused by active trigger points.

If the trigger points themselves are being caused, or are being aggravated and maintained, by poor posture, stressful work or leisure habits, unbalanced breathing patterns – or other lifestyle or controllable habits of use – then deactivating the trigger point will often only give short-term relief.

Of course, some trigger points exist for old, historic reasons, and there are no present habits to deal with, just a quick and safe deactivation of these troublesome facilitated areas.

But for many patients, removing or changing the underlying, ongoing, background of 'stress' (biomechanical, psychological and/or biochemical) should be a major focus of attention, to help to prevent a return of symptoms.

For people whose patterns of use are obviously creating, or aggravating, their health problems it makes sense to adopt a viewpoint that says that relief and improvement will only be achieved if the causes are removed, or if the person (or the part of the person that's in trouble) improves the ability to handle the ongoing stresses.

See Chapters 1 and 2 for discussion of adaptation processes.

This way of seeing health problems can be summarized as: 'lighten the load', and/or 'improve function to handle the load better'.

Rehabilitation aims to return the individual toward a state of normality that has been lost through trauma or ill health.

Rehabilitation features might include:

- normalization of soft tissue dysfunction, including abnormal tension and fibrosis, using methods such as massage, NMT, MET, MFR, PRT and/or articulation,
mobilization and/or other stretching procedures, such as yoga
- deactivation of myofascial trigger points, possibly involving massage, NMT, MET, MFR, PRT, spray and stretch, and/or articulation/mobilization
- or, appropriately trained and licensed practitioners might use injection or acupuncture in order to deactivate trigger points
- strengthening weakened structures, involving exercise and methods such as Pilates
- proprioceptive reeducation using physical therapy methods (e.g. wobble board, balance retraining, etc.) and spinal stabilization exercises, as well as methods such as those devised by Feldenkrais (1972), Hanna (1988), Pilates (Latey 2001, Knaster 1996), Trager (1987), and others
- postural and breathing reeducation, using physical therapy approaches as well as Alexander, yoga, tai chi and other similar systems
- ergonomic, nutritional and stress reeducation and management strategies, as appropriate to the individual
- psychotherapy, counseling or pain management techniques, such as cognitive behavior therapy
- occupational therapy, which specializes in activating healthy coping mechanisms, determining functional capacity, increasing activity and developing adaptive strategies to return the person to a greater level of self-reliance and quality of life
- appropriate exercise strategies to overcome deconditioning (Liebenson 1996).

You know which of these methods and elements are within your scope of practice, and/or your skill base.

For access to those that are not, appropriate referral is called for.

Example

Physical therapist, Dinah Bradley (1999), has described how to 'treat' trigger points by removing or reducing the stresses that caused them.

When patients with breathing pattern disorders are being assessed, she identifies trigger points in their intercostal muscles.

She uses an algometer (see Chapter 5) to assess and record how much pressure is required to produce the patient's pain when these points are compressed.

She then teaches better breathing methods, for home application.

When patients return to be reassessed, she retests the trigger points.

Box 7.10   Education/rehabilitation and self-help – *cont'd*

If their threshold has risen (that is more pressure is now needed to cause pain) she knows that there has been progress in rehabilitation of the breathing pattern.

The patient has been doing his home-work!

On the other hand, if pain thresholds are the same or have dropped (less pressure needed to cause the pain when pressed), she suspects that either home-work rehabilitation exercises have not been done regularly, or that other factors (greater emotional stress, for example) are current.

The same type of progress in pain threshold will be seen when trigger points calm down if overuse and/or postural stresses (and/or psychological stresses) are reduced or removed.

A formula for better health (and reduced trigger point activity)

- Lighten the adaptive load, or help to find ways to improve the person's ability to handle that load – whatever it is.
- Better breathing, better posture, better 'use of the self', reformed habits of sleep, exercise, stress coping and nutrition, will all achieve these objectives.

Resources

Self-help books that offer different approaches to enhanced levels of musculoskeletal wellbeing, include:

- *Modern Pilates* (Latey 2001). This describes clearly, and with abundant illustration, safe and effective strength, mobility and stability approaches based on Pilates methodology.
- *Maintaining Body Balance, Flexibility and Stability* (Chaitow 2004). This offers self-help advice using a range of methods (compression, muscle energy, positional release) as well as rehabilitation and improved breathing approaches. It recommends that home-care advice from the book should be used together with the advice and/or supervision of a licensed practitioner or therapist.
- Texts such as the excellent *Facilitated Stretching* (McAtee & Charland 1999) and *Stretching* (Anderson 1984) offer effective and safe methods for maintaining flexibility, as long as the advice given is followed closely, and excessive stretching is avoided.

CLINICAL NOTE

Key points from Chapter 7

1. There are many ways of deactivating myofascial trigger points.

2. Some trigger points may be functional, acting to support or stabilize unstable areas. Particular care should be taken before removing such support in hypermobile individuals (or joints).

3. Research confirms that the most effective methods involve compression – see Box 7.1 (also known as ischemic compression, inhibitory pressure and acupressure) and 'spray and stretch' methods (see Box 7.2).

4. Combinations of different physical methods (compression, damp heat, stretching, etc.) work well together in trigger point deactivation (Hou et al 2002).

5. Neuromuscular technique (or neuromuscular therapy) – NMT – uses all these methods, most of which derive from traditional forms of massage, both Western and Oriental (see also Box 7.6).

6. The evidence for manipulation as a treatment for trigger point activity is not strong, although benefits are reported when combined with other manual (soft tissue) methods.

7. Whatever treatments are used to deactivate trigger points, these are likely to recur unless the causes that produced them are removed, whether these relate to overuse, poor posture, poor breathing patterns, emotional factors, nutritional imbalances, hormonal disturbance or anything else. See Box 7.10.

References

Anderson B 1984 Stretching. Shelter, Bolinas, CA

Bailey M, Dick L 1992 Nociceptive considerations in treating with counterstrain. Journal of the American Osteopathic Association 92:334–341

Baldry P 1993 Acupuncture, trigger points and musculoskeletal pain. Churchill Livingstone, Edinburgh, p 91–103

Ballantyne F et al 2003 Effect of MET on hamstring extensibility: the mechanism of altered flexibility. Journal of Osteopathic Medicine 6(2):59–63

Barnes J 1996 Myofascial release in treatment of thoracic outlet syndrome. Journal of Bodywork and Movement Therapies 1(1):53–57

Barnes M F 1997 The basic science of myofascial release: morphologic change in connective tissue. Journal of Bodywork and Movement Therapies 1(4):231–238

Bowles C 1981 Functional technique – a modern perspective. Journal of the American Osteopathic Association 80(3):326–331

Bradley D 1999 In: Gilbert C (ed) Breathing retraining advice from three therapists. Journal of Bodywork and Movement Therapies 3(3):159–167

Cantu R, Grodin A 1992 Myofascial manipulation. Aspen Publications, Gaithersburg, MD

Chaitow L 1994 Integrated neuromuscular inhibition technique. British Journal of Osteopathy 13:17–20

Chaitow L 2001 Muscle energy techniques, 2nd edn. Churchill Livingstone, Edinburgh

Chaitow L 2003a Positional release techniques, 2nd edn. Churchill Livingstone, Edinburgh

Chaitow L 2003b Modern neuromuscular techniques, 2nd edn. Churchill Livingstone, Edinburgh

Chaitow L 2004 Maintaining balance, flexibility and stability. Churchill Livingstone, Edinburgh

Chaitow L, DeLany J 2000 Clinical applications of neuromuscular technique. Churchill Livingstone, Edinburgh

Chatchawan U, Thinkhamrop B, Kharmwan S et al 2005 Effectiveness of traditional Thai massage among patients with back pain associated with myofascial trigger points. Journal of Bodywork and Movement Therapies (Accepted for publication 2005)

Chikly B 1997 Lymph drainage therapy. Study guide level II. Chikly and UI Publishing, Florida

Chikly B 1999 Clinical perspectives: breast cancer reconstructive rehabilitation. Journal of Bodywork and Movement Therapies 3(1):11–16

Dardzinski J, Ostrov B, Hamann L 2000 Myofascial pain unresponsive to standard treatment. Successful use of a strain and counterstrain technique with physical therapy. Journal of Clinical Rheumatology 6(4):169–174

Davies C 2001 The trigger point therapy workbook. New Harbinger Publications, Oakland, CA

de las Peñas C-F 2004 Manual therapies in myofascial trigger point treatment: a systematic review. Journal of Bodywork and Movement Therapies 9(1):27–34

Deig D 2001 Positional release technique. Butterworth-Heinemann, Boston

Dorland's medical dictionary 1985 26th edn. W B Saunders, Philadelphia

Feldenkrais M 1972 Awareness through movement. Harper and Row, New York

Foldi M, Strossenreuther R 2005 Foundations of manual lymph drainage, 3rd edn. Elsevier Mosby, St Louis

Fritz S 1998 Mosby's basic science for soft tissue and movement therapies. Mosby, St Louis

Fryer G, Hodgson L 2005 The effect of manual pressure release on myofascial trigger points in the upper trapezius muscle. Journal of Bodywork and Movement Therapies (in press)

Gam A, Warming S, Larsen L 1998 Treatment of myofascial trigger points with ultrasound combined with massage and exercise – a randomised controlled trial. Pain 77:73–79

Greenman P 1996 Principles of manual medicine, 2nd edn. Williams & Wilkins, Baltimore

Haas M, Groupp E, Kraemer D 2004 Dose–response for chiropractic care of chronic low back pain. Spine Journal 4(5):574–583

Hanna T 1988 Somatics. Addison-Wesley, New York

Hanten W P, Barret M, Gillespie-Plesko M 1997 Effects of active head retraction with retraction/extension and occipital release on the pressure pain threshold of cervical and scapular trigger points. Physiotherapy Theory and Practice 13(4):285–291

Hanten W, Olsen S, Butts N et al 2000 Effectiveness of a home program of ischaemic pressure followed by sustained stretch for treatment of myofascial trigger points. Physical Therapy 80:997–1003

Harris R Piller N 2004 Three case studies indicating effectiveness of MLD on patients with primary and secondary lymphedema. Journal of Bodywork and Movement Therapies 7(4):213–222

Hong C-Z 1994 Considerations and recommendations regarding myofascial trigger points. Journal of Musculoskeletal Pain 2(1):29–59

Hoover H 1969 Collected papers. Academy of Applied Osteopathy Yearbook, Carmel, California

Hou C-R, Tsai L-C, Cheng K-F et al 2002 Immediate effects of various physical therapeutic modalities on cervical myofascial pain and trigger-point sensitivity. Archives of Physical Medicine and Rehabilitation 83:1406–1414

Hurwitz E, Morgenstern H, Harber P et al 2002 A randomized trial of medical care with and without physical therapy and chiropractic care with and without physical modalities for patients with low back pain: 6-month follow-up outcomes from the UCLA low back pain study. Spine 27:2193–2204

Jacobson E 1989 Shoulder pain and repetition strain injury. Journal of the American Osteopathic Association 89:1037–1045

Janda V 1989 Muscle function testing. Butterworths, London

Jones L 1981 Strain and counterstrain. Academy of Applied Osteopathy, Colorado Springs

Knaster M 1996 Discovering the body's wisdom. Bantam, New York

Kuchera M, McPartland J 1997 Myofascial trigger points. In: Ward R (ed) Foundations of osteopathic medicine. Williams & Wilkins, Baltimore

Latey P 2001 Modern Pilates. Allen & Unwin, NSW, Australia

Lewit K 1999 Manipulation in rehabilitation of the motor system, 3rd edn. Butterworths, London

Lewit K, Olsanska S 2004 Clinical importance of active scars: abnormal scars as a cause of myofascial pain. Journal of Manipulative and Physiological Therapeutics 27(6):399–402

Liebenson C 1989 Active muscular relaxation techniques (part 1). Journal of Manipulative and Physiological Therapeutics 12(6):446–451

Liebenson C 1990 Active muscular relaxation techniques (part 2). Journal of Manipulative and Physiological Therapeutics 13(1):2–6

Liebenson C 1996 Integrating rehabilitation into chiropractic practice. In: Liebenson C (ed) Rehabilitation of the spine. Williams & Wilkins, Baltimore

Mattes A 1995 Active isolated stretching. Privately published, Sarasota, FL

McAtee R, Charland J 1999 Facilitated stretching, 2nd edn. Human Kinetics, Champaign, IL

McPartland J 2004 Travell trigger points – molecular and osteopathic perspectives. Journal of the American Osteopathic Association 104(6):244–249

McPartland J M, Klofat I 1995 Strain und Counterstrain-Technik Kursunterlagen. Landesverbände der Deutschen Gesellschaft für Manuelle Medizin, Baden

Melzack R, Wall P (eds) 1994 Textbook of pain, 3rd edn. Churchill Livingstone, London, p 201–224

Mennell J 1974 Therapeutic use of cold. Journal of the American Osteopathic Association 74(12)

Mock L 1997 Myofascial release treatment of specific muscles of the upper extremity (levels 3 and 4). Clinical Bulletin of Myofascial Therapy 2(1):5–23

Oyama I, Rejba A, Lukban J et al 2004 Modified Thiele massage as therapeutic intervention for female patients with interstitial cystitis and high-tone pelvic floor dysfunction. Urology 64(5):862–865

Prateepavanich P, Kupniratsaikul V, Charoensak T 1999 The relationship between myofascial trigger points of gastrocnemius muscle and nocturnal calf cramps. Journal of the Medical Association of Thailand 82:451–459

Preyde M 2000 Effectiveness of massage therapy for subacute low-back pain: a randomized controlled trial. Canadian Medical Association Journal 162:1815–1820

Rachlin I 1994 Therapeutic massage in the treatment of myofascial pain syndromes and fibromyalgia. In: Rachlin E S (ed) Myofascial pain and fibromyalgia; trigger point management. Mosby, St Louis, p 455–472

Shea M 1993 Myofascial release – a manual for the spine and extremities. Shea Educational Group, Juno Beach, FL

Simons D 1987 Myofascial pain syndrome due to trigger points. In: Goodgold J (ed) Rehabilitation medicine. Mosby, St Louis, p 686–723

Simons D 2002 Understanding effective treatment of myofascial trigger points. Journal of Bodywork and Movement Therapies 6(2):81–88

Simons D, Travell J, Simons L 1999 Myofascial pain and dysfunction: the trigger point manual. Vol 1, The upper extremities, 2nd edn. Williams & Wilkins, Baltimore, MD

Trager M 1987 Mentastics. Station Hill, Mill Valley, CA

Travell J 1942 Technic for reduction and ambulatory treatment of sacroiliac displacement. Archives of Physical Therapy 23:222–232

Travell J 1952 Ethyl chloride spray for painful muscle spasm. Archives of Physical Medicine 33:291–298

Travell J, Simons D 1983 Myofascial pain and dysfunction: the trigger point manual. Vol 1, The upper extremities. Williams & Wilkins, Baltimore, MD

Twomey L, Taylor J 1982 Flexion, creep, dysfunction and hysteresis in the lumbar vertebral column. Spine 7(2):116–122

Van Buskirk R 1990 Nociceptive reflexes and the somatic dysfunction. Journal of the American Osteopathic Association 90:792–809

Ward R (ed) 1997 Foundations of osteopathic medicine. Williams & Wilkins, Baltimore

Weiss J 2001 Pelvic floor myofascial trigger points: manual therapy for interstitial cystitis and the urgency-frequency syndrome. Journal of Urology 166:2226–2231

Zink J 1981 The posterior axillary folds – a gateway for osteopathic treatment of the upper extremities. Osteopathic Annals 9(3):81–88

CHAPTER EIGHT

Integrating trigger point application into massage

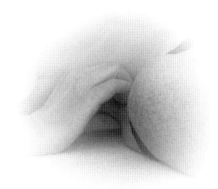

INTRODUCTION

The information in the book up to this point has involved both theory and descriptions of methodology specifically focused on understanding, assessing for, determining appropriateness of treatment to, and finally treatment approaches for, trigger points.

Only small modifications to conventional therapeutic massage are necessary to effectively identify and treat most trigger points. There are many benefits for both client and therapist in the integration of trigger point treatment methods into massage.

In fact, a majority of the methods used to assess for, and treat, trigger points are aspects of massage methodology, which incorporates many of the features needed to provide an integrated approach to trigger point treatment including:

- ischemic compression
- skin manipulation
- management of edema
- encouraging circulation and stretching
- reduction in sympathetic arousal.

The tools of trigger point treatment are therefore already, literally, in the therapist's hands. What is required is a greater knowledge of the role of trigger points in causing symptoms; how to locate them, and how to integrate existing knowledge into a usable formula for managing myofascial pain.

Important issues for the massage therapist include:

- learning to become aware of trigger point activity by considering aspects of massage as assessment
- making good clinical decisions about whether the person should be referred for more comprehensive evaluation because the trigger point activity may involve some sort of organ dysfunction, or may be related to a protective mechanism
- becoming skilled in evaluation and clinical reasoning to discern if the trigger point activity is serving some useful purpose and whether or not it is appropriate to treat (deactivate) a trigger point
- deciding which trigger points to treat for the best outcomes.
- incorporating trigger point assessment and treatment into the massage so that the generalized full body experience of the massage is not compromised.

Previous chapters have addressed many aspects of these issues. This chapter specifically concerns itself with the integration of trigger point theory, assessment and treatment into the massage application. Massage as a system is malleable and can easily accommodate inclusion of many different soft tissue approaches such as manual treatment of trigger points.

To summarize:

- Massage is the manual manipulation of the soft tissues.
- Trigger points can be identified and treated using soft tissue manipulation techniques.
- Soft tissue manipulations create various mechanical forces and neuroendocrine stimuli.

QUALITIES OF TOUCH

Massage application involves touching the body to manipulate the soft tissue, influence body fluid movement and stimulate neuroendocrine responses.

How the physical contact is applied is considered the *quality of touch*.

All massage consists of a combination of the following qualities of touch:

- *Depth of pressure* (compressive force), which can be light, moderate, deep, or variable. Depth of pressure is extremely important. Most soft tissue areas of the body consist of three to five layers of tissue, including: the skin; the superficial fascia; the superficial, middle, and deep layers of muscle; and the various fascial sheaths and connective tissue structures. Pressure must be delivered through each successive layer to reach the deeper layers without damage and discomfort to the more superficial tissues. The deeper the pressure, the broader the base of contact required on the surface of the body. It takes more pressure to address thick, dense tissue than delicate thin tissue (Fig. 8.1). Depth of pressure is important for both assessment and treatment of trigger points. Trigger points can form in all layers of tissue, and in order to treat these you have to be able to apply the correct level of pressure to both reach the location of the point, as well as compress the tissue to alter flow of circulation. Obviously

trigger points located in surface tissue require less depth of pressure when being treated than those located in deeper muscle layers.

- *Drag* is the amount of pull (stretch) on the tissue (tensile force) (Fig. 8.2). Drag is applicable for various types of palpation assessment for trigger points including skin drag assessment and functional technique to identify areas of ease and bind – as discussed in earlier chapters. Drag is also a component of myofascial release methods used to treat trigger points.
- *Direction* can move from the center of the body out (centrifugal) or in from the extremities toward the center of the body (centripetal). It can proceed from proximal to distal (or vice versa) of the muscle, following the muscle fibers, transverse to the tissue fibers, or in circular motions. Direction is a factor in stretching tissues containing trigger points or in the methods that influence blood and lymphatic fluid movement (Fig. 8.3).
- *Speed* of manipulations can be fast, slow or variable. Trigger point assessment is usually in the moderate to slow speed range, while treatment speed can be variable.
- *Rhythm* refers to the regularity of application of the

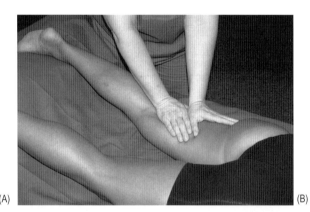
(A)

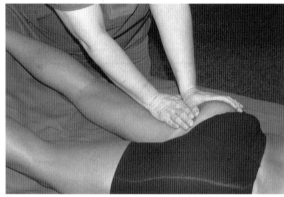
(B)

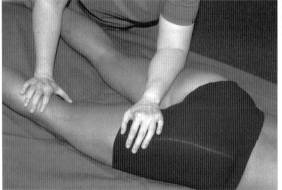
(C)

Figure 8.1   Depth of pressure. A: light; B: moderate; C: deep. (Reproduced with kind permission from Mosby's Massage Career Development Series, 2006.)

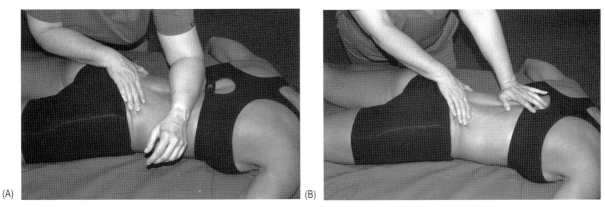

Figure 8.2   Drag. (Reproduced with kind permission from Mosby's Massage Career Development Series, 2006.)

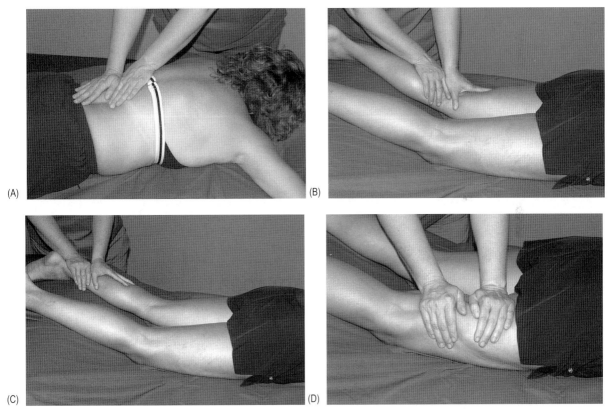

Figure 8.3   Direction. A: Centrifugal; B: centripetal; C: distal to proximal; D: transverse. (Reproduced with kind permission from Mosby's Massage Career Development Series, 2006.)

technique. If the method is applied at regular intervals, it is considered even, or rhythmic. If the method is disjointed or irregular, it is considered uneven, or non-rhythmic. The on/off aspect of compression applied to a trigger point to encourage circulation to the area is applied in a rhythmic manner. Lymphatic drain application is also, ideally, rhythmic.

- *Frequency* is the rate at which the method repeats itself in a given time frame. This aspect of massage relates to how often the treatment method, such as ischemic compression, is repeated when treating trigger points. In general, the massage practitioner repeats each method about three times before moving or switching to a different approach. The first application is assessment, the second is treatment, and the third is post assessment. If the post assessment indicates remaining dysfunction, then the frequency is increased to repeat the treatment/post assessment a couple more times.

- *Duration* is the length of time that the method lasts, or that the manipulation stays in the same location. Typically, duration should not be more than 60 seconds although functional methods can be an exception and may be applied for longer periods. Duration relates to how long compression is applied to trigger points, or how long a stretch is held.

Example

The following example describes how these qualities of the touch influence massage methods used to treat trigger points.

Let us imagine that lymphatic drainage methods are indicated in the management and treatment of a patient's trigger points. Lymphatic drainage application can be explained as follows: light pressure, with mild drag of the skin, in a slow rhythmic manner, directed toward the closest major drainage area. The application is repeated multiple times for a duration of 3–5 minutes.

More on qualities of touch

Through these varied qualities of touch, simple massage methods are adapted to the desired outcomes for the client. These qualities of touch provide the therapeutic benefit. The mode of application (e.g. gliding, kneading, compression) provides the most efficient application. Each method can be varied, depending on the desired outcome, by adjusting depth, drag, direction, speed, rhythm, frequency and duration.

In perfecting massage application, it is the *quality of touch* that is important, arguably more so than the

method. Quality of touch is altered when there is a contraindication or caution for massage.

As examples:
- when a person is fatigued, often the duration of the application is reduced
- if a client has a fragile bone structure, the depth of pressure is altered
- if someone is agitated, the rhythm can be modified to create a relaxing effect.

COMPONENTS OF MASSAGE APPLICATION RELEVANT TO TRIGGER POINT ASSESSMENT AND TREATMENT

Providing a meaningful therapeutic massage is dependent on the therapist's ability to execute the various movements associated with massage in ways that are relevant to the patient's condition and needs.

Using efficient body mechanics is another consideration, since massage involves manual labor and can be potentially stressful for the therapist.

Incorporating trigger point assessment and treatment requires an awareness of both how to do this efficiently, and why it is being done.

THE EFFECTS OF MASSAGE

All massage manipulations introduce forces into the soft tissues. These forces produce a variety of physiological responses.

Some massage applications are more mechanical than others, and connective tissue and fluid dynamics are most affected by mechanical force.

- Connective tissue is influenced by mechanical forces by changing its pliability, orientation and length.
- The movement of fluids in the body involves mechanical processes, so that forces applied to the body can mimic various pumping mechanisms of the heart, arteries, veins, lymphatics, muscles, respiratory system and digestive tract (Lederman 1997).
- Neuroendocrine stimulation (involving hormones and the nervous system) occurs when forces are applied during massage that generate various shifts in physiology (Ernst & Fialka 1994).
- Massage causes the release of vasodilator substances which then influence circulation in an area (Tiran 2000), reducing sympathetic autonomic nervous system dominance (De Domenico & Wood 2000).
- Massage stimulates the relaxation response, reducing sympathetic autonomic nervous system dominance (De Domenico & Wood 2000).

- Forces applied during massage stimulate proprioceptors which have the ability to alter motor tone in muscles (Lederman 1997).

It is easy to understand how mechanical force application can be used to address trigger point activity. Typically these two responses to massage – involving circulation and connective tissue – occur together, although the intent of the massage application can be to target one response more than the other.

It is helpful to identify the different types of mechanical forces and to understand the ways in which mechanical forces applied during massage act therapeutically on the body to address trigger points.

The forces created by massage are tension loading, compression loading, bending loading, shear loading, rotation or torsion loading, and combined loading.

Tension loading (Fig. 8.4)

Tension forces (also called tensile force) occur when two ends of a structure are pulled apart from one another. Tension force is created by methods such as traction, longitudinal stretching, and stroking with tissue drag. Tissues elongate under tension loading with the intent of lengthening shortened tissues. Tension loading is also effective in moving body fluids. Tension force is used during massage with applications that drag, glide, lengthen and stretch tissue to elongate connective tissues and lengthen short muscles. Gliding and stretching make the most use of tension loading.

The distinguishing characteristic of gliding strokes is that they are applied horizontally in relation to the tissues, generating a tensile force.

When applying gliding strokes, light pressure remains on the skin. Moderate pressure extends through the subcutaneous layer of the skin to reach muscle tissue but not so deep as to compress the tissue against the underlying bony structure. Moderate to heavy pressure that puts sufficient drag on the tissue mechanically affects the connective tissue and the proprioceptors (spindle cells and Golgi tendon organs) found in the muscle. Heavy pressure produces a distinctive compressive force of the soft tissue against the bone.

Strokes that use moderate pressure from the fingers and toes toward the heart following the muscle fiber direction are excellent for mechanical and reflexive stimulation of blood flow, particularly venous return and lymphatics. Light to moderate pressure with short, repetitive gliding following the patterns for the lymph vessels is the basis for manual lymph drainage.

Compression loading (Fig. 8.5)

Compressive forces occur when two structures are pressed together.

Compression moves down into the tissues, with varying depths of pressure adding bending and compressive forces. Compressive force is a component of massage application that is described as depth of pressure. The manipulations involving compression usually penetrate the subcutaneous layer, whereas in the resting position they stay on the skin surface. Excess compressive force could potentially rupture or tear muscle tissue, causing bruising, microtrauma and connective tissue damage. This is a concern when pressure is applied to deeper layers of tissue (see Chapter 6).

To avoid tissue damage, the massage therapist should distribute the compressive force of massage over a broad contact area on the body. Therefore, the more compressive force being used to either assess or

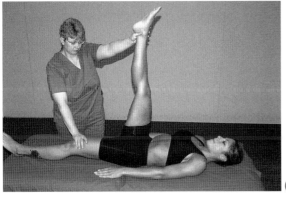
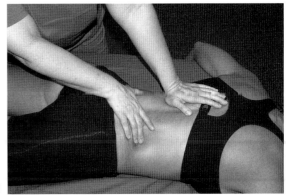

(A)   (B)

Figure 8.4   Tension. A: Stretching; B: gliding stroking with drag. (Reproduced with kind permission from Mosby's Massage Career Development Series, 2006.)

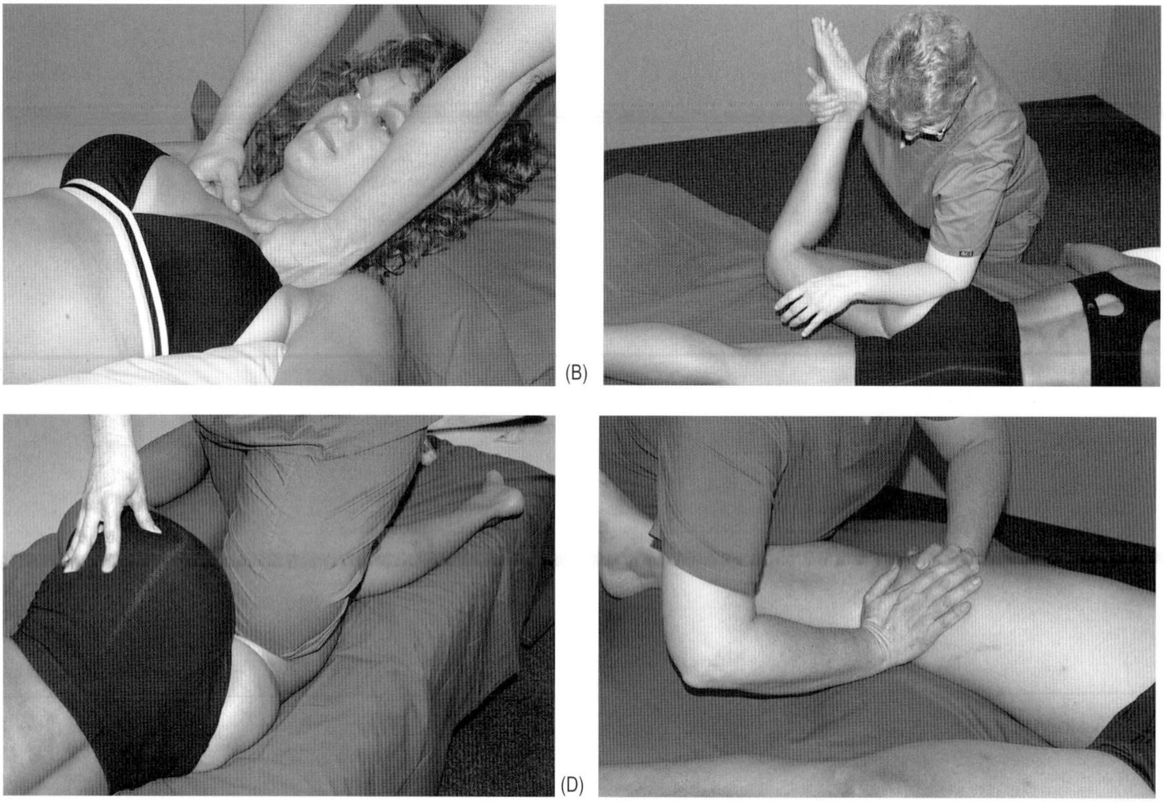

Figure 8.5   Compression. (Reproduced with kind permission from Mosby's Massage Career Development Series, 2006.)

treat the tissue, the broader the base of contact with the tissue, in order to prevent injury.

Compressive force is used therapeutically to affect circulation, nerve stimulation and connective tissue pliability. Compression is effective when used in a rhythmic pump-like way, to facilitate fluid dynamics. Tissue will shorten and widen, increasing the pressure within the tissue and affecting fluid flow, and is therefore an excellent method for enhancing circulation. The pressure against the capillary beds changes the pressure inside the vessels and encourages fluid exchange. Compression appropriately applied to arteries allows back pressure to build, and when the compression is released, it encourages increased arterial flow.

Much of the effect of compression results from pressing tissue against the underlying bone, causing it to spread. Sustained compression will result in more pliable connective tissue structures and is effective in reducing tissue density and binding. Compression loading is a main method used in trigger point treatment.

Bending loading (Fig. 8.6)

Bending forces are a combination of compression and tension. One side of a structure is exposed to compressive forces while the other side is exposed to tensile forces. Bending occurs during many massage applications. Pressure is applied to the tissue, or force is applied across the fiber, or across the direction of the muscles, tendons or ligaments, and fascial sheaths.

Assessing for trigger points by lifting tissue involves a bending force, as does the pincer method of treating trigger points. Bending forces are excellent for direct stretching of tissue containing trigger points and for increasing connective tissue pliability and affecting proprioceptors in the tendons and bellies of the muscles.

A variation of the lifting manipulation is skin rolling. Applying deep bending forces attempts to lift the muscular component away from the bone, but skin rolling lifts only the skin from the underlying fascial and muscle layer. This has a warming and softening effect on the superficial fascia, causes reflexive stimulation of the spinal nerves, and is an excellent assessment method for

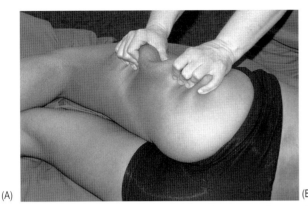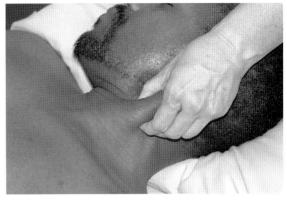

(A)   (B)

Figure 8.6   Bending. (Reproduced with kind permission from Mosby's Massage Career Development Series, 2006.)

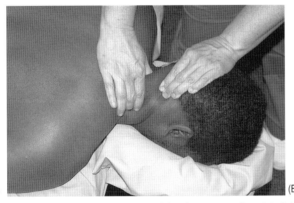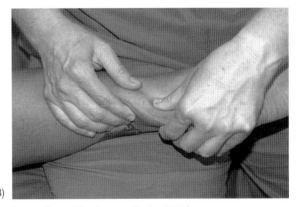

(A)   (B)

Figure 8.7   Shear. (Reproduced with kind permission from Mosby's Massage Career Development Series, 2006.)

trigger points. Areas of 'stuck' skin often suggest underlying problems (see Chapter 6).

Shear loading (Fig. 8.7)

Shear forces move tissue back and forth, creating a combined pattern of compression and elongation of tissue. Shearing is a sliding force. As a result, significant friction is created between the structures that are sliding against each other, which damages tissues. This type of damage is often called microtrauma. Microtrauma predisposes the musculotendinous junction to inflammatory problems, connective tissue changes, adhesion and attachment trigger points (see Chapter 3).

The massage method of friction uses shear force to generate physiological changes by increasing connective tissue pliability, so ensuring that tissue layers slide over one another instead of adhering to underlying layers creating *bind*.

Shear loading application also assists in pain reduction through the gate control mechanisms of counterirritation and hyperstimulation analgesia (Kolt & Snyder-Mackler 2003).

Friction consists of small, deep movements performed on a local area, providing shear force to the tissue. Friction manipulation prevents and breaks up local adhesions in connective tissue, especially over tendons, ligaments and scars.

This method is not used over an acute injury or fresh scar, and should only be used if the adaptive capacity of the client can respond to superimposed tissue trauma. Since excess friction (shearing force) from movement or injury may result in an inflammatory irritation that causes many soft tissue problems, therapeutic application of friction to a trigger point is a potential treatment, especially if the trigger point is close to connective tissue changes such as a scar. Using friction to address trigger point activity is not as common as other methods. Friction will increase blood flow to an area but can also cause edema from the resulting inflammation and tissue damage.

Simons et al (1999) caution against use of friction near muscle attachments as inflammatory responses are likely (enthesitis).

The movement in friction is usually transverse to the fiber direction and is generally performed for 30 seconds to 10 minutes.

The result of this type of friction is usually initiation of a small, controlled inflammatory response. The chemicals released during inflammation result in activation of tissue repair mechanisms with reorganization of connective tissue. This type of work, coupled with proper healing and rehabilitation, can be very valuable.

As the tissue responds to the friction, it is often useful to gradually begin to stretch the area and increase the pressure. The sensation for the client may be intense, and if it is painful, the application should be modified to a tolerable level so that the client reports the sensation as a 'good hurt'.

The recommended way to work within the client's comfort zone is to use pressure sufficient for him or her to feel the specific area but not complain of pain. Friction should be continued until the sensation diminishes. Gradually increase the pressure until the client again feels the specific area. Begin friction again and repeat the sequence for up to 10 minutes.

The area being frictioned may be tender to the touch for 48 hours after use of the technique. The sensation should be similar to a mild after-exercise soreness. Because the focus of friction is the controlled application of a localized inflammatory response, heat and redness are caused by the release of histamine. The area should not bruise.

Rotation or torsion loading (Fig. 8.8)

This force type is a combined application of compression and wringing, resulting in elongation of tissue along the axis of rotation. It is used where a combined effect on both fluid dynamics and connective tissue pliability is desired.

Torsion forces are best thought of as twisting forces.

Massage methods that use kneading introduce torsion forces as soft tissue is lifted, rolled and squeezed. The main purpose of this manipulation is to lift tissue, applying bend, shear and torsion forces. Torsion force can be used as a therapeutic force that affects connective tissue in the body. Kneading soft tissue can identify trigger points by assessing changes in tissue texture and can be an aspect of treatment, especially as an aspect of stretching tissue or encouraging circulation or fluid movement in soft tissue.

Changes in depth of pressure and drag determine whether the kneading manipulation is perceived by the client as superficial or deep. By the nature of the manipulation, the pressure and pull peak when the tissue is lifted to its maximum and decrease at the beginning and end of the manipulation.

Combined loading (Fig. 8.9)

Combining two or more forces effectively loads tissue. The more forces applied to tissue the more intense the response.

Tension and compression underlie all the different modes of loading; therefore, any form of manipulation is either tension, compression or a combination of these.

Tension force is important in conditions where tissue needs to be elongated, and compression force

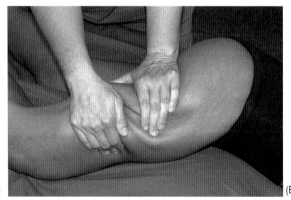
(A)

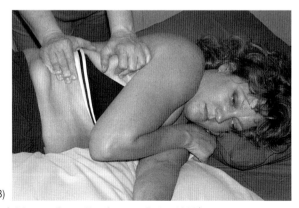
(B)

Figure 8.8   Torsion. (Reproduced with kind permission from Mosby's Massage Career Development Series, 2006.)

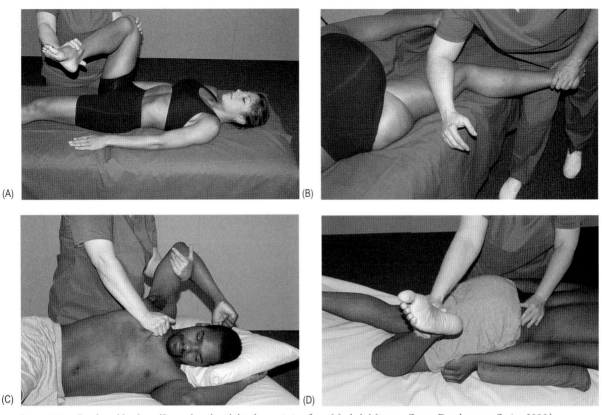

(A)   (B)   (C)   (D)

Figure 8.9   Combined loading. (Reproduced with kind permission from Mosby's Massage Career Development Series, 2006.)

where fluid flow needs to be affected. Because tissues housing trigger points need to be stretched a tension force would be used during the treatment trigger points.

JOINT MOVEMENT METHODS

- Joint movement can be used for trigger point assessment and treatment.
- Joint movement is used to position muscles for muscle energy methods and stretching tissues containing trigger points.
- Joint movement also encourages fluid movement in the lymphatic, arterial and venous circulation systems.
- Much of the pumping action that moves these fluids in the vessels results from rhythmic compression during joint movement and muscle contraction.
- The tendons, ligaments and joint capsule are warmed by joint movement, and this mechanical effect helps keep these tissues pliable.

Types of joint movement methods

Joint movement involves moving the jointed areas within the physiologic limits of range of motion of the client. The two basic types of joint movement used in massage therapy are active and passive.

Active joint movement means that the client moves the joint by active contraction of muscle groups.

The two variations of active joint movement are as follows:

1. Active assisted movement, which occurs when both the client and the massage practitioner move the area (Fig. 8.10).
2. Active resistive movement, which occurs when the client actively moves the joint against a resistance provided by the massage practitioner (Fig. 8.11).

Passive joint movement occurs when the client's muscles stay relaxed and the massage practitioner moves the joint with no assistance from the client (Fig. 8.12).

Since muscle energy techniques are focused on specific muscles or muscle groups, it is important to be

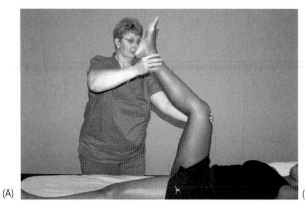
(A)

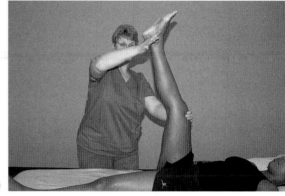
(B)

Figure 8.10   Active assisted movement. (Reproduced with kind permission from Mosby's Massage Career Development Series, 2006.)

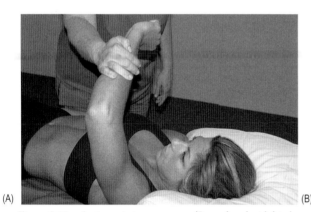
(A)

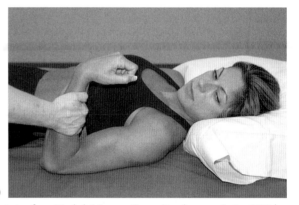
(B)

Figure 8.11   Active resistive movement. (Reproduced with kind permission from Mosby's Massage Career Development Series, 2006.)

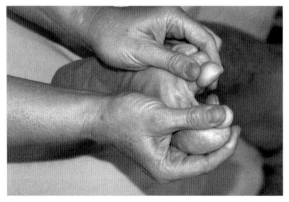

Figure 8.12   Passive joint movement. (Reproduced with kind permission from Mosby's Massage Career Development Series, 2006.)

able to position muscles so that the muscle attachments are either close together or in a lengthening phase with the attachments separated, and joint movement is how this positioning is accomplished.

Failure to lengthen and stretch the area containing trigger points results in the eventual return of the original symptoms. Muscle energy approaches are more effective than passive stretching in achieving the proper response.

Joint movement is effective for positioning tissues to be stretched. Muscles that are nearer the surface respond to joint movement to position them, but this method is less effective for the small deep muscles. Trigger points located in deep layers of muscle or in a muscle that is difficult to lengthen by moving the body are addressed with local bending, shearing and torsion to lengthen and stretch the local area.

MASSAGE AND PREVENTION OF TRIGGER POINTS

Massage may be one of the most effective prevention measures for trigger point development, as explained below.

- Massage can address causal factors preventing the formation of trigger points.
- General full body massage that incorporates application to the various tissue types and layers of soft tissue may help to shift the circulation and metabolic dysfunction to a more normal state.
- Muscles with the tendency to form trigger points can be maintained in a more pliable and lengthened state through the use of massage.
- The soft tissue are regularly searched for changes during general massage and the soft tissue can be normalized before the trigger point develops or the surrounding tissues become fibrotic, and before satellite points form.
- Massage can also help maintain a more normal breathing pattern and autonomic nervous system balance by inducing relaxation.
- For massage to be effective the person would need to have a thorough massage on a regular basis – with weekly sessions ideal and at the minimum, monthly.

BASIC MASSAGE PROTOCOL WITH SUGGESTIONS FOR ASSESSING FOR AND TREATING TRIGGER POINTS (Boxes 8.1 and 8.2)

The protocol outlined is only one example of how to assess for and treat trigger points during an integrated general massage application.

As this protocol is practiced, the massage therapist should become familiar with how the assessment and treatment of trigger points is woven into the concept of a full body relaxation massage. Once there is an understanding of the concepts involved, the process should become easy to modify and adapt to best fit the individual style of the massage therapist.

Face and head

- Massage of the face is relaxing; therefore, if the face is treated first, it can set the stage for a calming massage, or if the face is treated at the end of the session, it will gently finish the massage.
- Lightly and systematically stroke the face in multiple directions, assessing for temperature and tissue texture changes that might indicate trigger point activity (Fig. 8.13).

Box 8.1 Sequence of massage based on clinical reasoning to achieve specific outcomes

1. Massage application intent (outcome) determines mode of application and variation in quality of touch:
   - mode of application – influenced by type/mode of application (glide, knead, oscillation compression, percussion, movement, etc.)
   - quality of touch – location of application, depth of pressure (light to deep), tissue drag, rate (speed) of application, rhythm, direction, frequency (number of repetitions) and duration of application of the method
2. mode of application with variations in quality of touch generate:
3. mechanical forces (tension, compression, bend, shear, torsion) to effect tissue changes from physical loading leading to:
4. influence on physiology:
   - mechanical changes (tissue repair, connective tissue viscosity and pliability, fluid dynamic)
   - neurological changes (stimulus response-motor system and neuromuscular, pain reflexes, mechanoreceptors)
   - psycho-physiological changes (changes in mood, pain perception, sympathetic and parasympathetic balance)
   - interplay with unknown pathways and physiology (energetic, meridians, chakras, etc.)
5. contribute to development of treatment approach
6. resulting in desired outcomes.

- To assess for the possible presence of trigger points, move the skin systematically into ease and bind (ease: the way it moves the most; bind: the way it moves the least). Areas of bind may indicate trigger point activity. To increase circulation in the area of bind move the skin into multiple directions of ease, and hold the ease position for up to 30–60 seconds. This method may be sufficient to address trigger points in this area.
- Address the muscle structures. Light to moderate compressive force is adequate to address the area. The muscles of mastication often house trigger points. Hold the tissues housing the trigger point in its ease direction, using bending forces, and then move the tissues into bind to stretch the area.
- If active trigger points remain after the above methods have been applied, then use a combination of compression on points combined with a

Box 8.2   General suggestions for incorporating trigger points into the massage (Simons et al 1999)

- Trigger points in the belly of muscles are usually located in short, concentrically contracted muscles.
- Trigger points located near the attachments are usually found in eccentric patterns and in long, inhibited, muscles acting as antagonists to concentrically contracted muscles.
- Generally it is best to treat central (belly) points first, as removing their influence often deactivates the attachment points in the same muscle.
- Do not overtreat trigger points.
- Only address the trigger points that recreate the symptoms the client is experiencing.
- Remember anything can feel like a trigger point if pressed on hard, for long enough.
- Only address the trigger points that are most painful, most medial, and most proximal, and that also recreate the client's symptoms.
- Leave the rest alone and monitor them over the course of three or four massage sessions to identify improvement.
- When posture and function improve and/or normalize with regular massage, trigger points will often go away on their own.
- Contracted muscles containing trigger points may be serving useful purposes, possibly as a response to instability.
- It is best to address the trigger point activity in shortened (hypertonic, contracted) tissues first and wait to see if the trigger points in the 'lengthened (weak) muscles', and at the attachments, resolve as posture and muscle interaction normalizes.
- To balance the long inhibited muscles, the following strengthening procedures can be used.
  Isometric contraction: The muscle is placed in a specific position within its range and the client contracts against resistance, without any actual movement taking place. This is particularly useful in maintaining strength in a muscle that cannot be exercised normally, due to dysfunction in its associated joint. The strengthening effect is greatest in the middle and inner range of movement.
  Concentric movements: This is the most common type of muscle-strengthening activity and involves the contraction and shortening of a muscle by taking it through its active range of movement with a weighted resistance. For example, the biceps muscle concentrically

Box 8.2   – cont'd

contracts when lifting a weight, by flexing the elbow. Movements should be made slowly to develop control throughout the contraction range. Sudden, quick contractions can lead to injury and are likely to increase muscle tension by overstimulating the nerve receptors.

A muscle produces its greatest force in the mid-range. If the muscle is only strengthened in the mid-range, it will only function in that range and may become chronically short. So it is important always to include exercises with light resistance through the fullest range of both concentric and eccentric contraction to develop both strength and length.

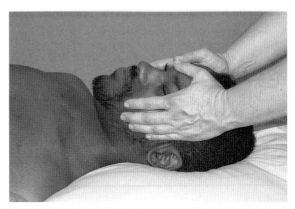

Figure 8.13   Massage of the face and head. (Reproduced with kind permission from Mosby's Massage Career Development Series, 2006.)

rhythmic on (5 seconds)/off (3 seconds) pressure, for about 10 repetitions.
- In the areas where trigger points have been addressed, the tissues housing the trigger points need to be lengthened. Use gliding and gentle kneading to stretch the areas.
- To finish massaging the face, return to the initial light stroking of the lymphatic drainage style to support fluid exchange in the area.
- General massage of the head begins with the assessment process for potential trigger points.
- Typically hair prevents using skin drag palpation methods. However, the scalp can be moved into ease and bind positions, and the muscles can be palpated for trigger point symptoms (pain, etc.).
- Any trigger points identified that are appropriate to treat during the massage are most easily addressed

with compression methods, and then manually stretched using ease and bind movement of the scalp in a myofascial release approach.

- Some clients enjoy having their hair gently stroked and pulled during massage and pulling large bunches of the hair in a slow steady manner stretches the tissues to which it attaches.
- Compression applied to the sides of the head, and to the front and back, coupled with a scratching motion to the scalp can be very pleasant, and at the same time allows assessment for the presence of trigger points (Fig. 8.14).

Neck

- Address this area with the client prone and/or side-lying.
- Systematically, lightly stroke the area. Then increase the pressure slightly and slowly move the tissue into ease and bind.
- Include assessment methods of scanning for heat and skin drag.
- Identify any potential areas of trigger point activity to be further addressed.
- Use gliding with a compressive element beginning at the middle of the back of the head at the trapezius attachments, and slowly drag the tissue to the distal attachment of the trapezius at the acromion process and lateral third of the clavicle. Slow the speed of the glide and increase pressure over the areas that may be housing trigger points to confirm if there are active points that meet the criteria for treatment (Fig. 8.15).
- With the client prone, begin again at the head and glide toward the acromion. When the area of a

trigger point is located, cease gliding and apply compression. Muscle energy methods can also be used (contraction followed by stretch).

- Then reverse the direction and work from distal to proximal, applying tension force to stretch the area (Fig. 8.16).
- Next knead and glide across the muscle fibers, making sure that bending, shear and torsion forces are only sufficient to create a pleasurable sensation while assessing for changes in the tissues housing the previously treated trigger point.
- Increase intensity of the kneading to further stretch the local tissue in the trigger point area, and then again apply tension force – this time by passively or actively using joint movement and stretching the area.
- Gentle, rocking, rhythmic range of motion of the area (oscillation) may be used to continue to relax the area.

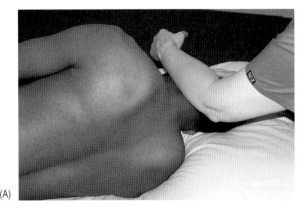
(A)

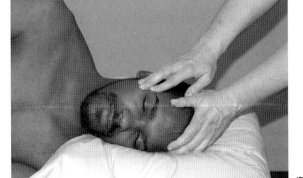

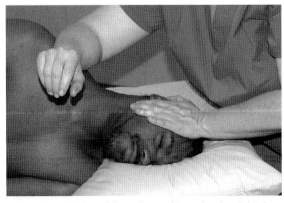
(B)

Figure 8.14 Post assessment of the head. (Reproduced with kind permission from Mosby's Massage Career Development Series, 2006.)

Figure 8.15 Gliding of the neck area. (Reproduced with kind permission from Mosby's Massage Career Development Series, 2006.)

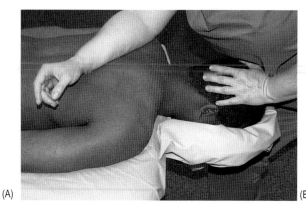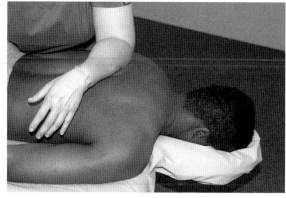

(A)   (B)

Figure 8.16   Gliding prone. A: Proximal to distal; B: distal to proximal. (Reproduced with kind permission from Mosby's Massage Career Development Series, 2006.)

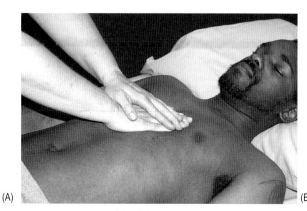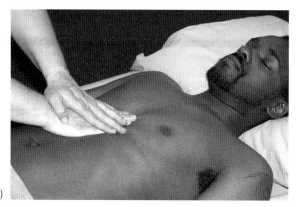

(A)   (B)

Figure 8.17   Treatment of trigger point using ease and bind positioning. A: Ease; B: bind. (Reproduced with kind permission from Mosby's Massage Career Development Series, 2006.)

Torso anterior

- When massaging this area, breathing mechanisms may be influenced. The massage therapist affects breathing by maintaining soft tissue mobility in the area and helping to encourage balance between sympathetic and parasympathetic autonomic nervous system function. This is generally accomplished with a relaxation focus from the general massage.
- The following muscles in this area are specifically targeted for massage because they tend to shorten during breathing dysfunction and commonly house trigger points:
  scalenes
  sternocleidomastoid
  serratus anterior
  upper trapezius
  pectoralis major and minor
  abdominals
  psoas.

- The intercostals and diaphragm, which are the major breathing muscles, are also addressed.
- Massage begins superficially and progresses to deeper tissue layers and then finishes off with superficial work again. During the massage, assessment for trigger point activity occurs – for example any time that tissues being massaged appear denser or tenser than they should, pressure (compression) into them may demonstrate trigger point activity if the patient reports symptoms that he or she is familiar with. ('That's the pain I have been experiencing.')
- In general, to treat trigger points as the massage progresses, hold the tissue in ease position until release is felt, or for up to 60 seconds. The tissues should then be moved into bind using myofascial approaches to stretch the tissue (Fig. 8.17).
- Use gliding with a compressive element beginning at the shoulder and work from the distal attach-

ment of the pectoralis major at the arm toward the sternum following fiber direction. This can be done in supine or side-lying position with the client rolled (Fig. 8.18).

- Repeat three or four times, each time increasing the drag and moving more slowly.
- When the area of a trigger point is located, cease gliding and apply compression.
- Muscle energy methods can also be used (have the patient contract the muscle isometrically, then stretch).
- Positional release methods are especially effective in this area (press the point, then position the tissues to remove the discomfort caused by compression, and hold for a minute or so) (Fig. 8.19).
- Then reverse the direction and work from distal to proximal, applying tension force to stretch the area.
- Knead and glide across the muscle fibers, making sure that bending, shear and torsion forces are only sufficient to create a pleasurable sensation while

assessing for changes in the tissues housing the previously treated trigger point (Fig. 8.20).
- Increase the intensity of the kneading to further stretch the local tissue in the trigger point area and then again apply tension force, this time by passively or actively using joint movement and stretching the area if possible (Fig. 8.21).
- Work with each area as needed as it becomes convenient during the general massage session. Use the least invasive measures possible to deactivate trigger points, and restore a more normal muscle resting length.
- It is likely that if the breathing has been dysfunctional for an extended period of time (over 3 months) connective tissue changes have occurred.
- Focused connective tissue massage application may be useful and effective. Once the soft tissue is more normal, then gentle mobilization of the thorax is appropriate.

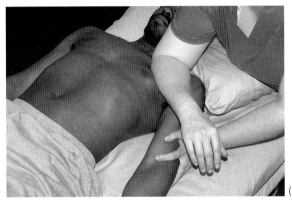

(A)

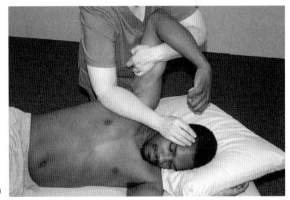

(B)

Figure 8.18   Gliding with compression. A: Supine; B: side-lying. (Reproduced with kind permission from Mosby's Massage Career Development Series, 2006.)

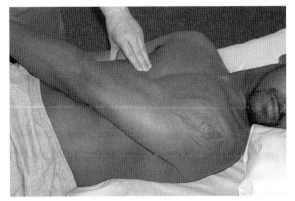

Figure 8.19   Positional release. (Reproduced with kind permission from Mosby's Massage Career Development Series, 2006.)

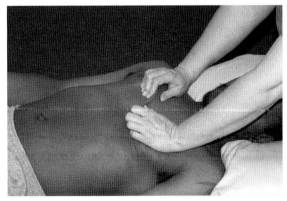

Figure 8.20   Bending and torsion to assess trigger point. (Reproduced with kind permission from Mosby's Massage Career Development Series, 2006.)

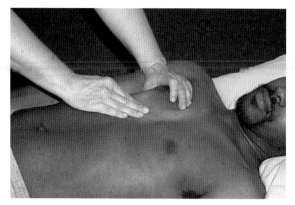

Figure 8.21 Bending to stretch trigger point area. (Reproduced with kind permission from Mosby's Massage Career Development Series, 2006.)

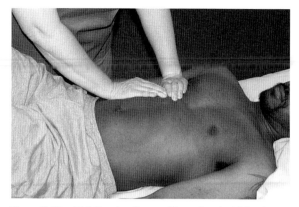

Figure 8.22 Mobilize the rib cage. (Reproduced with kind permission from Mosby's Massage Career Development Series, 2006.)

- If the thoracic vertebrae and ribs are restricted, chiropractic or other joint manipulation methods may be appropriate and referral is indicated.
- The massage therapist can use functional techniques, for example moving the tissues into ease and bind, in order to increase the mobility of the area.
- Gently move the rib cage with broad-based compression. Assess for areas that move easily and those that are restricted (Fig. 8.22). Identify the amount of rigidity in the ribs with the client supine by applying compression to the thorax beginning near the clavicles and moving down toward the lower ribs, maintaining compressive force near the costal cartilage.
- Compression against the lateral aspect of the thorax with the client in a side-lying position will assess rib mobility in both facet and costal joints.
- Begin applying the compression near the axilla and then move down toward the lower ribs.
- Sufficient force needs to be used while applying the compression to feel the ribs spring but not so much to cause discomfort.
- Normal responses would be provided by a feeling of equal mobility bilaterally.
- A feeling of stiffness or rigidity indicates immobility.
- Identify the areas of most mobility and the areas of most restriction.
- Position the client so that a broad-based compressive force can be applied to the areas of ease – the most mobile.
- Gently and slowly apply compression until the area begins to bind.
- Hold this position and have the client cough.
- Coughing will act as a muscle energy method and also support mobility of the joint through activation of the muscles. Repeat three or four times.

- Gently mobilize the entire thorax with rhythmic compression.
- Reassess the area of most bind/restriction. If the areas treated have improved, then a different area is located and the sequence is repeated.
- Next, palpate for trigger points in the intercostals, pectoralis minor and anterior serratus.
- Clients are not always tolerant to this, so be reassuring, direct and precise.
- Use positional release to release these points by moving the client or having them move into various positions until the pain in the tender point decreases (Fig. 8.23).
- Apply local tissue stretching to tissues housing trigger points, using gliding and kneading.
- Move to the abdomen and knead slowly across the fiber direction, assessing for trigger point activity, and then determine appropriateness of treatment, based on the history and outcome goals.
- Skin drag palpation is often ticklish in this area so is not used, but scanning for areas of excess heat (or coolness) is possible, and can be useful.
- The psoas muscles should be assessed and treated for trigger points at this time.
- Rhythmic compression to the entire anterior torso area stimulates the lymphatic flow and blood circulation and encourages relaxed breathing.

Posterior torso

- This area can be addressed in prone or side-lying. It frequently becomes involved if there are breathing function difficulties.
- The muscles commonly housing trigger points are:
  serratus posterior, superior and inferior
  levator scapulae
  rhomboids

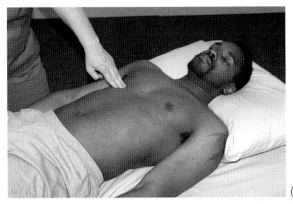

(A)

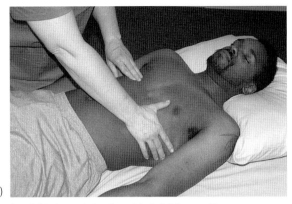

(B)

Figure 8.23 Positional release of intercostal trigger point. (Reproduced with kind permission from Mosby's Massage Career Development Series, 2006.)

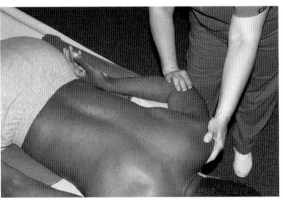

(A)

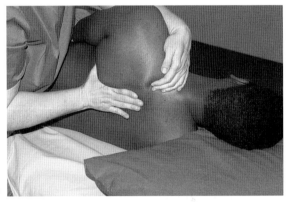

(B)

Figure 8.24 Addressing surface tissue layers. (Reproduced with kind permission from Mosby's Massage Career Development Series, 2006.)

latissimus dorsi
erector spinae and paraspinals
quadratus lumborum.

- As described previously, massage begins superficially and progresses to deeper layers and then finishes off with superficial work (Fig. 8.24).
- It is helpful to place the client so that the surface layer of tissue is in a slack position by placing the attachments of the muscle close together and propping the client in this position, so that they can remain relaxed. In some situations, the side-lying position may be better for this.
- Begin with skin drag palpation and scanning to assess for possible trigger point activity.
- Use gliding with a compressive element, beginning at the iliac crest and working diagonally along the fibers of latissimus dorsi, ending at the axilla.
- Repeat three or four times, each time increasing the drag and moving more slowly to address deeper tissue layers.

- Identify areas of tissue bind, heat, increased histamine response and muscle 'knots' (Fig. 8.25).
- Move up to the thoracolumbar junction and repeat the same sequence on the lower trapezius.
- Then begin near the tip of the shoulder and glide toward the middle thoracic area to address the middle trapezius. Repeat three or four times, increasing drag and decreasing speed.
- Begin again near the acromion and address the upper trapezius with one or two gliding strokes to complete the surface area (Fig. 8.26).
- Choose which trigger points are appropriate for treatment. When the area of the trigger point is located, cease gliding and apply compression (Fig. 8.27).
- Muscle energy methods can also be used (Fig. 8.28).
- Then, reverse the direction and work from distal to proximal, applying tension force to stretch the area.
- Knead and glide across the muscle fibers, making sure that bending, shear and torsion forces do not

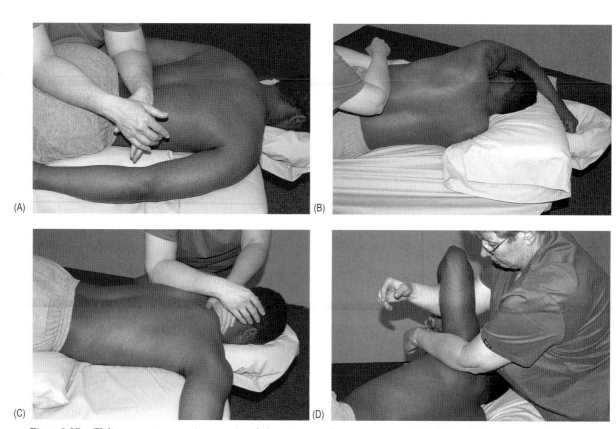

(A)   (B)   (C)   (D)

Figure 8.25   Gliding posterior torso. A: prone; B: side-lying. Reverse direction. C: prone; D: side-lying. (Reproduced with kind permission from Mosby's Massage Career Development Series, 2006.)

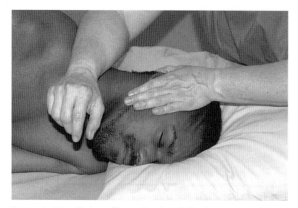

Figure 8.26   Gliding. (Reproduced with kind permission from Mosby's Massage Career Development Series, 2006.)

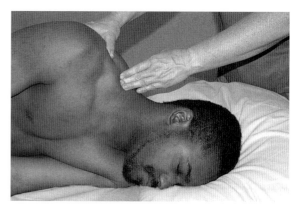

Figure 8.27   Identify trigger point and treat with compression. (Reproduced with kind permission from Mosby's Massage Career Development Series, 2006.)

create unpleasant sensations, while assessing for changes in the tissues housing any previously treated trigger point.

- Increase intensity of the kneading to further stretch the local tissue in the trigger point area and then again apply tension force, this time by passively or actively using joint movement and stretching the area (Fig. 8.29).

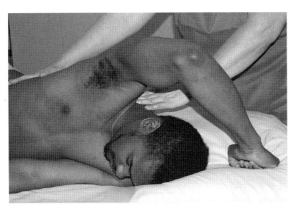

Figure 8.28   Treating trigger point with muscle energy technique. (Reproduced with kind permission from Mosby's Massage Career Development Series, 2006.)

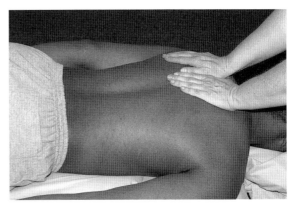

Figure 8.30   Applying compression near facet joints. (Reproduced with kind permission from Mosby's Massage Career Development Series, 2006.)

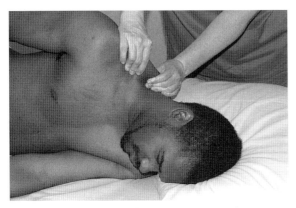

Figure 8.29   Using bend and torsion forces to stretch trigger point area. (Reproduced with kind permission from Mosby's Massage Career Development Series, 2006.)

- Knead the area again to increase circulation to the area and shift nervous system responses.
- Move the skin into multiple directions of ease, and holding the ease position for up to 30–60 seconds. If appropriate, use lymphatic drainage methods in the area.
- Gentle, rocking, rhythmic ranges of motion of the area (oscillation) may be used to continue to relax the area.
- Identify rigidity in the ribs with the client prone bilaterally (on both sides of the spine) at the facet joints, beginning near the seventh cervical vertebra and moving down toward the lower ribs maintaining compressive force near the facet joints (Fig. 8.30).
- If an area is identified, assess the area for trigger point activity and treat with integrated muscle energy technique.

- Rhythmic compression to the area stimulates various aspects of fluid movement, supports relaxed breathing and finishes the massage of the area.

Shoulder, arm and hand

- The area is massaged in supine, prone, side-lying and seated positions. Massage of the torso and neck naturally progresses to the shoulder, arm and hand (Fig. 8.31).
- Commencing with client prone, massage begins superficially, progresses to deeper layers and then finishes off with superficial work.
- Finish massaging the area with kneading, compression and gliding.
- During the general massage, tissue is assessed for trigger point activity relating to any symptoms the client may have. All assessment methods can be incorporated into the massage application.
- Before applying ischemic compression methods, use less invasive methods such as positional release (moving tissues into 'ease'), which often successfully deactivates the trigger point if followed by light stretching.
- To increase circulation to the area, and shift nervous system responses, move the skin into multiple directions of ease, and holding the ease position for up to 30–60 seconds.
- Then move the tissue into bind to stretch the area.
- If trigger point activity remains, combine compression with passive movements of the arm.
- Stretch the area with either active or passive joint movement or direct tissue application, incorporating gliding and kneading whichever is more effective. It is also appropriate to use a combination of stretching methods (Fig. 8.32).

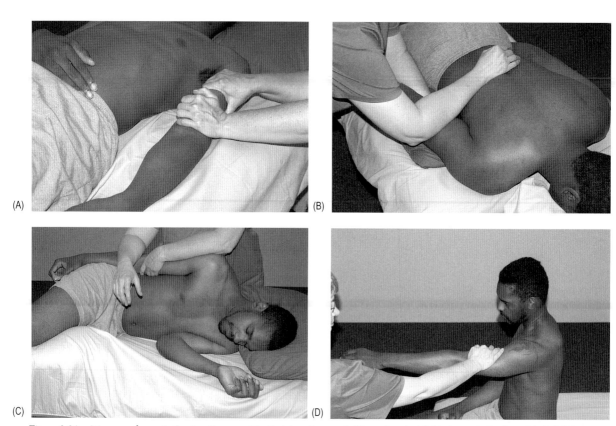

(A)   (B)   (C)   (D)

Figure 8.31 Massage of arm. A: Supine; B: prone; C: side-lying; D: seated. (Reproduced with kind permission from Mosby's Massage Career Development Series, 2006.)

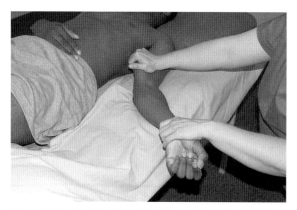

Figure 8.32 Combined stretching, biceps. (Reproduced with kind permission from Mosby's Massage Career Development Series, 2006.)

- The intrinsic muscles of the hand are addressed next.
- Systematically work the area, using compression and gliding of the soft tissue between the fingers, the web of the thumb, and on the palm that opposes the thumb and little finger.
- Trigger point activity responds to compression methods or positional release and direct tissue stretching.
- There is also a network of lymphatic vessels in the palm that when rhythmically compressed assist lymphatic movement (Fig. 8.33).

Hip

- The hip is massaged in prone and side-lying positions. Massage of the torso naturally progresses to the hip.
- Massage begins superficially and progresses to deeper layers and then finishes off with superficial work.

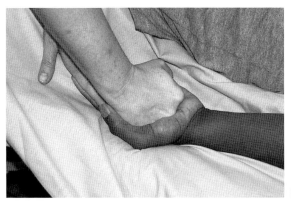

Figure 8.33 Compression of the hand. (Reproduced with kind permission from Mosby's Massage Career Development Series, 2006.)

- Systematically, lightly stroke the area. This movement incorporates assessment for trigger point activity.
- To increase circulation to the area and shift nervous system responses, move the skin into multiple directions of ease, and hold the ease position for up to 30–60 seconds (Fig. 8.34).
- Methods of lymphatic drainage are also appropriate if edema is present.
- Increase the pressure slightly. Begin posteriorly to address the lumbar region that connects with the hip.
- This area was addressed while massaging the torso but now is massaged in relationship to the hip. Carry the strokes into the gluteus maximus (Fig. 8.35).
- Use gliding with a compressive element and glide toward the hip.
- Repeat with strokes on latissimus dorsi again, in relationship to hip function. Begin at the shoulder and carry the stroke all the way into the opposite gluteus maximus (Fig. 8.36).
- Systematically repeat the gliding, interspersing with kneading to assess the deeper tissue layers for trigger point symptoms or the tell-tale knots that refer pain in trigger point patterns.
- If trigger points are identified, address with the least invasive method of skin ease and bind movement or skin rolling.
- Progress to compression methods with positional release. As a last resort, if there are connective tissue changes, shear forces introduced with friction can be used (Fig. 8.37).

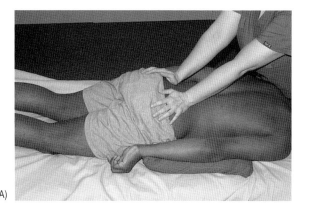

(A)

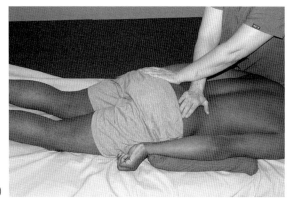

(B)

Figure 8.34 Moving skin in multiple directions on the hip area. (Reproduced with kind permission from Mosby's Massage Career Development Series, 2006.)

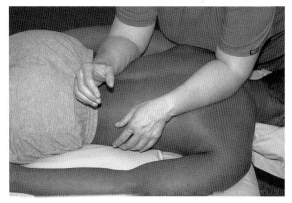

Figure 8.35 Massage connecting stroke from lumbar to hip. (Reproduced with kind permission from Mosby's Massage Career Development Series, 2006.)

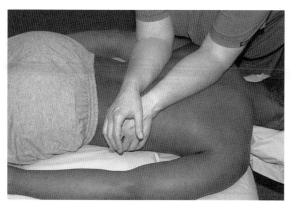

Figure 8.36 Massage using tension force for latissimus and opposite gluteus maximus. (Reproduced with kind permission from Mosby's Massage Career Development Series, 2006.)

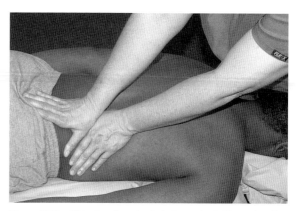

Figure 8.38 Skin drag lymphatic drain method. (Reproduced with kind permission from Mosby's Massage Career Development Series, 2006.)

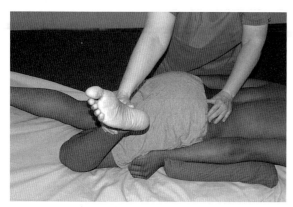

Figure 8.37 Compression combined with positional release on trigger point near sacroiliac joint. (Reproduced with kind permission from Mosby's Massage Career Development Series, 2006.)

- Stretch the area with direct tissue methods by kneading and slow gliding and myofascial methods.
- Lymphatic drainage methods support fluid movement in the area (Fig. 8.38).
- Finish by gliding and kneading the entire area.

Thighs, legs and feet

- The area can be massaged in all basic positions: supine, prone, side-lying and seated.
- Massage of the area naturally progresses from the hip.
- As with other body regions, massage begins superficially, progresses to deeper layers and then finishes off with superficial work.
- To increase circulation to the area and influence nervous system responses, move the skin in mul-

tiple directions of ease, and hold the ease position for up to 30–60 seconds.
- Increase the pressure slightly and again introduce gliding and kneading of the entire area.
- Systematically repeat the gliding, interspersing with kneading to assess the deeper tissue layers for trigger point symptoms or the tell-tale knots that refer pain in trigger point patterns (Fig. 8.39).
- If trigger points are identified, address them with the least invasive method of skin ease and bind movement or skin rolling.
- Progress to compression methods with positional release.
- As a last resort, if there are connective tissue changes, shear forces introduced with friction can be used.
- Stretch the area with direct tissue methods by kneading and slow gliding and myofascial methods (Fig. 8.40).
- Move the hip and knee passively through flexion, extension, internal and external rotation to assess for restrictions in joint function.
- Trigger point activity can be addressed with compression and muscle energy methods (Fig. 8.41).
- Move the hip and knee passively through flexion, extension, internal and external rotation stretching as appropriate, in relationship to trigger point treatment.
- Lymphatic drainage methods support fluid movement in the area.
- Finish by gliding and kneading the entire area.
- Add gentle shaking and oscillation in various positions.
- The intrinsic muscles of the foot are addressed next.
- Systematically work using compression and gliding of the soft tissue of the sole of the foot.

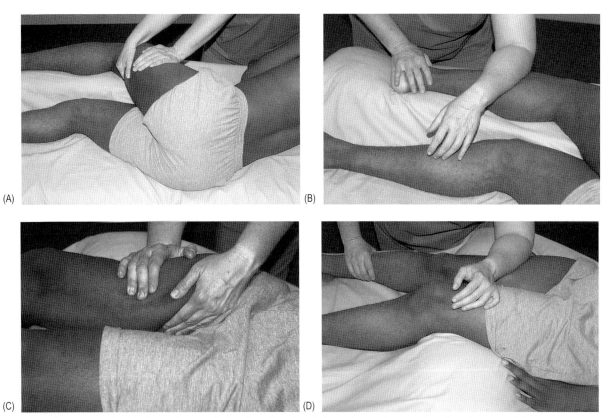

Figure 8.39   Massage of thigh and leg. A: Side-lying kneading; B: side-lying gliding; C: supine kneading; D: supine gliding. (Reproduced with kind permission from Mosby's Massage Career Development Series, 2006.)

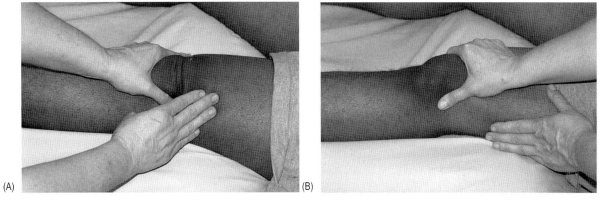

Figure 8.40   Identification of trigger point and treatment with compression. A. Assess with skin drag; B: treat with broad-based compression. (Reproduced with kind permission from Mosby's Massage Career Development Series, 2006.)

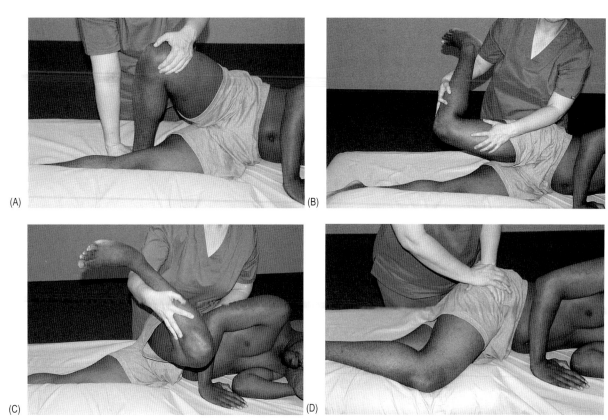

Figure 8.41   Joint movement assessment with compression treatment of trigger point. A: Range of motion – external rotation; B: range of motion – internal rotation; C: range of motion – flexion with internal rotation; D: treatment with broad-based compression. (Reproduced with kind permission from Mosby's Massage Career Development Series, 2006.)

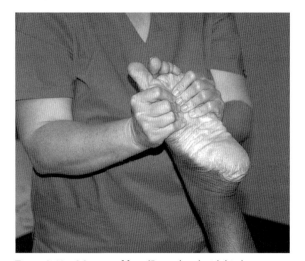

Figure 8.42   Massage of foot. (Reproduced with kind permission from Mosby's Massage Career Development Series, 2006.)

- There is also a network of lymphatic vessels in the sole of the feet that, when rhythmically compressed, will assist lymphatic movement (Fig. 8.42).
- Treat trigger points as appropriate.
- To finish off, use gentle shaking and oscillation and compression and passive movement.

The protocol outlined above is just one example of how massage and trigger point assessment and treatment efficiently combine with massage.

It is suggested that the reader follow the protocol as presented a few times to grasp the concept, and then adapt the methods to best fit their individual style and client needs.

MASSAGE AS SPOT (LOCAL) TREATMENT FOR TRIGGER POINTS

It is also appropriate for massage therapists to assess for, and treat, trigger points using soft tissue methods without performing a full body massage application.

It is common for massage to be used for spot (local) treatment.

Including trigger point assessment and treatment as an aspect of targeted massage, in a specific area, is effective.

The chair massage approach can be enhanced by incorporating trigger point work into the session.

Chair massage often focuses on the neck, shoulders and back – which are all common areas for trigger point development.

Usually this massage approach is performed over clothing and uses compression as the primary method, therefore targeting the compressive force on active trigger points, followed by stretching.

All this is easily incorporated into the chair massage.

Assessment is more difficult since direct contact with the skin is limited.

Therefore trigger point activity needs to be identified while the tissue is being compressed or kneaded during the basic massage, before compressive force is specifically focused to address the trigger point.

After this, the area is stretched either with joint movement or by kneading or bending the tissue directly.

CLINICAL NOTE

Key points from Chapter 8

1. Trigger point assessment and treatment can easily and effectively be integrated into massage.

2. Massage easily adapts to include trigger point assessment and treatment.

3. Massage consists of application of mechanical forces applied to soft tissue.

4. Mechanical forces applied during massage can result in therapeutic benefits.

5. The relaxing nature of massage supports trigger point treatment.

6. Full body general massage with a relaxation outcome is not compromised by incorporating trigger point assessment and treatment, as long as specific outcomes are identified and the trigger point work specifically addresses these outcomes.

7. Previous chapters prepared the massage therapist for understanding and identifying trigger point activity and the information in those chapters can be used to make appropriate clinical decisions relating to treatment and the most effective type of treatment.

8. The protocol presented provides a format for the therapist to experience how massage can be used to assess for and treat trigger points.

9. Once the concept is grasped then it becomes efficient and effective for trigger point treatment to be a natural aspect of massage.

10. The massage therapist, with practice, can adapt this information for effective integration into any style of massage.

References

De Domenico G, Wood E 1997 Beard's massage, 4th edn. W B Saunders, Philadelphia

Ernst E, Fialka V 1994 The clinical effectiveness of massage therapy – a critical review. Forsch Komplementärmed 1:226–232

Kolt G S, Snyder-Mackler L (eds) 2003 Physical therapies in sport and exercise. Churchill Livingstone, Edinburgh

Lederman E 1997 Fundamentals of manual therapy: physiology, neurology, and psychology. Churchill Livingstone, Edinburgh

Simons D, Travell J, Simons L 1999 Myofascial pain and dysfunction, 2nd edn. Upper body. Williams & Wilkins, Baltimore

Tiran D 2000 Clinical aromatherapy for pregnancy and childbirth. Churchill Livingstone, Edinburgh

CHAPTER NINE

Non-manual trigger point deactivation methods

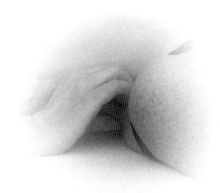

In Chapter 7 the main manual methods for deactivating trigger points were outlined in some detail.

It is important for therapists to have a clear understanding of other approaches to treatment of myofascial pain, and this chapter contains that information.

This chapter will include details of acupuncture, dry needling and injection methods, as well as microcurrent, ultrasound and metabolic (and nutritional) approaches.

There will also be brief summaries of the value or otherwise of TENS (transcutaneous electrical nerve stimulation) and laser treatment.

It is obviously essential that none of these methods is used unless the therapist is both trained and licensed to practice them.

It is, however, important that there is an understanding of what the methods involve and what evidence exists of their benefits, so that intelligent and informed advice can be offered to patients, and appropriate interdisciplinary referrals can be made where appropriate.

The following non-manual methods of trigger point deactivation are discussed in this chapter:

1. Acupuncture, dry needling and injection (Baldry 1993). See Box 9.1.
2. Laser treatment. See Box 9.2.
3. Magnetic treatment. See Box 9.3.
4. Metabolic rehabilitation (such as thyroid replacement) and nutrition (Lowe 1997, 2000, Lowe & Honeyman-Lowe 1998, Simons et al 1999). See Box 9.4.
5. Microcurrent applications (McMakin 1998). See Box 9.5.
6. Ultrasound (Lowe & Honeyman-Lowe 1998). See Box 9.6.
7. Topical creams, ointments and essential oils (McPartland 2004). See Box 9.7.
8. Hydrotherapy and watsu. See Box 9.8.

Box 9.1   Needles and injection treatment of trigger point pain

There are three main areas of trigger point treatment involving needles:

1. acupuncture
2. dry needling
3. injections.

Each of these will be explained below.

Even if you are never going to use a needle to treat trigger points (or anything else) it is important that you have an understanding of these methods because some patients/clients will certainly have experienced them, and some may ask advice regarding the possible usefulness of one or other of these treatment approaches. At the very least you should know what's involved, what the drawbacks might be, and the relative success rates.

Confusion and explanations
Before looking at these three needling variations it is necessary to clarify some confusion that can be summarized by the question, 'Are acupuncture points and trigger points the same?'

The answer seems to be – 'usually'.

Box 9.1   Needles and injection treatment of trigger point pain – *cont'd*

Before attempting to answer that question it is necessary to explain the difference between 'traditional' acupuncture points, and *ah shi* points.

- Traditional acupuncture points are located in precise anatomical sites, linked together in long lines, chains or meridians.
- Acupuncture point locations are easily confirmed by measuring electrical resistance of the skin, as briefly explained in Chapter 6.
- Figure 9.1 shows part of the gallbladder meridian of traditional acupuncture. Note how much the pathway of the meridian follows the pain distribution from an upper trapezius trigger point, as described in Chapter 6, and illustrated in Figure 6.17.
- Acupuncture points show signs of lowered electrical resistance because of increased water (hydrosis, sweat) that lowers skin resistance to electricity (Mann 1963).
- The importance of increased fluid in and under skin tissues near trigger points (probably because of increased sympathetic activity) was discussed in Chapter 6.
- The same additional skin changes (loss of elasticity) that occur in relation to trigger points also take place over and around acupuncture points (also discussed in Chapter 6).
- Not only are both sorts of points (acupuncture and trigger) detectable and sensitive, but they are also equally treatable, using manual pressure techniques, and what's more, they occupy more or less the same positions in at least 70% of cases (Melzack & Wall).

Are acupuncture points and trigger points the same?
- Pain researchers Melzack, Stillwell & Fox (1997), as well as Simons, Travell & Simons (1999), say that there is little, if any, difference between acupuncture points and most trigger points.
- Melzack & Wall (1989) have concluded that 'trigger points and acupuncture points, when used for pain control, although discovered independently and labeled differently, represent the same phenomenon'.
- Kawakita et al (2002) believe that there is no difference at all between acupuncture and trigger points, both being nothing more than sensitized neural structures (as discussed under the topic of sensitization and facilitation in Chapter 2).
- Not everyone agrees; for example, Baldry (1993) claims that there are differences in the make-up of acupuncture and trigger points.

Ah shi **points**
- In acupuncture treatment there are points, known as *ah shi* points, which are not listed on the traditional meridian maps, that are also treated.
- These are local areas that should not hurt when touched, but which do.
- They include all painful points that occur spontaneously, usually related to particular joint problems or disease.
- *Ah shi* points seem to be identical to the 'tender' points described by Jones (1981) in his strain/counterstrain positional release method (see Box 7.3) and also to active trigger points.

Three invasive trigger point treatment methods
NOTE: Acupuncture and dry needling techniques should only be used by fully trained and appropriately licensed therapists and practitioners.

1. Acupuncture
- Muscle pain has been treated using acupuncture for thousands of years. In the sixth century AD the Chinese physician Sun Ssu-Mo described how he treated muscular pain by inserting needles into tender (*ah shi*) points.
- Baldry (2002) says that about 10% of adults, and almost all children, with trigger point pain are 'strong responders'. With such individuals all that is needed is for an acupuncture needle to be inserted into the tissues overlying a trigger point, barely breaking the skin, and then withdrawn.

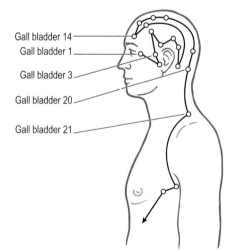

Gall bladder 14
Gall bladder 1
Gall bladder 3
Gall bladder 20
Gall bladder 21

Figure 9.1   Location of some important acupuncture points on the head and neck. Research indicates that over 75% of defined acupuncture points are also sites of common trigger points. (From Chaitow 2003.)

Box 9.1   Needles and injection treatment of trigger point pain – *cont'd*

- Because the therapist cannot know in advance if a person is a strong, average or weak responder, Baldry's approach is ideal as a first treatment.
- After the needle has been withdrawn the point is retested with compression to see whether the pain has reduced or vanished. If it has not responded to superficial needling, the next treatment involves the needle being inserted more deeply, and left in place for 30 seconds or more, before retesting.
- Weak responders, who fail to benefit from the 30-second needle retention, might have needles left in place for even longer, and/or rotated strongly, or stimulated with an electrical current.
- Baldry (2002) and others (Bowsher 1990) have given neurological explanations for the results of superficial needling.

2. Dry needling

- The first physician to use dry needling for the deactivation of trigger points, instead of acupuncture, was Karel Lewit in Czechoslovakia. Lewit (1979) reported this method after treating 241 patients with myofascial trigger point pain between 1975 and 1976.
- Since then thousands of practitioners have used 'dry needling' to deactivate trigger points.
- Practitioners who use dry needling usually perform a rapid series of insertions of the needle, into the trigger point, from different angles, attempting to provoke a number of twitch responses (Fig. 9.2).
- Hong (1994) has shown that dry needling, although sometimes successful in deactivating trigger points, commonly leads to bleeding in the tissues, as well as possible damage to local nerves. A severe deep aching

usually starts 2 to 8 hours after the treatment and lasts up to 24 hours. This sort of vigorous needling is only appropriate for very hardy individuals, and not at all suitable for frail or fragile patients.

Dry needling example
This example (below) of dry needling is taken from a research study by Ingber (2000) into treatment of shoulder problems.

Interestingly the treatment includes not only needling but both compression and stretching. It would be useful to know the results of compression and stretching alone, compared with the needling method described below:

Myofascial treatment is administered to the subscapularis muscle by dry needling or ischemic compression (myofascial massage), followed by carefully controlled stretching of the subscapularis.

The dry needling procedure to the subscapularis muscle is administered with the patient lying in the supine position with the arm supported by the plinth and positioned in 0° to 15° of internal rotation and 75° of abduction. The subscapularis trigger points are located by relaxing the patient while palpating for the most tender area in the posterior axillary wall, which is often located near the most superomedial aspect of the scapula. When radiating pain is noted by the patient [when compressed] the trigger point is dry-needled by rapidly peppering the site with a 'fast-in, fast-out' movement of a sterile acupuncture needle. The trigger point is needled until no further local twitch response is evoked by the needle movement. The arm is then immediately

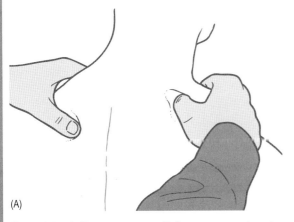
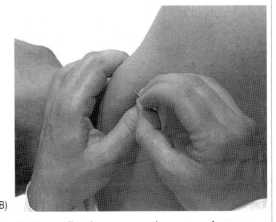

(A)   (B)

Figure 9.2   A: Pincer pressure applied to upper trapezius trigger point. B: Dry needling (or acupuncture) treatment of upper trapezius trigger point.

Box 9.1   Needles and injection treatment of trigger point pain – *cont'd*

taken through a full range of motion, abducting several times through an arc of 90° to 180° and back to 90°. ... After this the subscapularis trigger point is treated with myofascial massage or ischemic compression. Ischemic compression is performed by progressively increasing finger pressure at the trigger point to tolerance, which often evokes pain radiating to the trigger zone if the patient is properly relaxed.

Which is best, acupuncture or dry needling?
In one study Irnich et al (2002) showed that acupuncture was superior to dry needling in improving range of motion, and that it was better to use acupuncture at a distance from painful areas, rather than needling close to the pain.

Other studies suggest that that dry needling is better than acupuncture (Alvarez & Rockwell 2002).

A lot may depend on the practitioners using the particular methods, and their skills.

Some people react badly to most needling methods, especially if there are neurological imbalances and widespread disturbance of pain processing in the brain, such as exists in conditions such as fibromyalgia.

Such individuals may benefit from extremely light needle application (just a few seconds, barely breaking the skin; Baldry 2002), or they may be better off receiving one or other of the manual or alternative methods described in this chapter.

3. Injecting trigger points with pain-killing medication
Gupta et al (2003) tested the use of a combination of medications to inject trigger points (lidocaine, ketorolac (Toradol), and steroids); 47 patients diagnosed with active trigger points were treated with lidocaine alone, and 42 were treated with a combination of lidocaine, Toradol and steroid.

Patients were asked to chart their pain on a visual analogue scale (VAS – as described in Chapter 5) for 7 days.

The patients returned for 1- and 3-month check-ups.

Results showed that patients treated with a combination of lidocaine, Toradol and steroid had better pain control, needed fewer repeat injections, and had better resolution of symptoms than patients treated with lidocaine alone.

However, pain relief was only fully effective in 27% of those who received lidocaine, and in 39% of those who received the combination of medications as an injection.

These are not particularly impressive results!

Previous research has shown that dry needling had much the same effects as local anesthetic, corticosteroid and coolant spray in the treatment of lower back pain (Garvey et al 1989).

More recently Karakurum et al (2001) treated tension headache and found that muscle dry needling gave the same level of improvement in pain and neck range of motion as dummy (placebo) dry needling.

There are other studies that show better, and some that show poorer, results than these.

If there is benefit is it from the medication or the needling?
It seems reasonable to ask whether the benefits of injection derive from the drugs used, or the needling.

Some researchers have looked at the difference between injecting drugs such as lidocaine, and simple saline (salt water).

Many different medications have been used, and most of them give the same results as the injection of normal saline (salt water) (Frost et al 1980, Garvey et al 1989, Hameroff 1981).

When there is pain relief it lasts longer than would be expected from the medication alone.

This suggests that whatever is happening to ease pain, it is not just the medication effect, and that it may be the needle effect (as in the dry needling and acupuncture examples above).

Botox for trigger points?
A more recent innovation has been injection of botulinum toxin into trigger points. Some benefit has been shown in one study (Cheshire et al 1994) but in another study Botox was found to give the same benefit as salt water (Wheeler et al 1998).

Again it could be speculated that the needle was giving whatever pain relief was achieved rather than what was in the needle.

Conclusion
Acupuncture and dry needling appear to offer some benefits, but it is not clear to what extent associated soft tissue and stretching methods contribute to improvement.

Box 9.2   Laser treatment

Huguenin (2004) reviewed the use of laser treatment of myofascial pain, and says that there is poor evidence for the use of lasers of all types (low level, infrared, pulsed infrared, helium-neon, etc.) in treatment of trigger points.

Although some studies show some benefits (Olavi et al 1989), the evidence is not strong (Waylonis et al 1988).

Thorsen et al (1992) actually found that a dummy laser produced better results than a real laser when treating trigger points involved in neck and shoulder pain.

Conclusion

There appears to be little evidence of benefit from laser treatment of trigger point pain.

Box 9.3   Magnetic treatment

Research at the University of Tennessee into magnetic therapy appeared to show some benefit (Brown et al 2000).

For example, 60% of people with chronic pelvic pain, wearing active magnets (applied to abdominal trigger points), had 50% reduction in pain, compared with 33% wearing placebo magnets. The results suggest the longer magnets are used the better the effects. Much more research is needed to be conclusive, but research up to now seems to point to some benefit, and no risk or side effects.

An Italian study looking at the short- and medium-term effects of magnetic application in treatment of myofascial pain showed positive results.

- The equipment used was a *magnetic coil stimulator*, involving a similar process to that used to produce magnetic pulsations for an MRI scan.
- Eighteen patients with upper trapezius myofascial trigger points (TPs) received 10 magnetic stimulation treatments, of 20 minutes each.

- 4000 20 Hz magnetic pulsations were administered, in 5-second bursts, at the trigger point.
- Other patients received placebo (dummy) treatment to the trigger points, from a non-functioning ultrasound therapy device.
- Patients were assessed before treatment, at the end of treatment, and again 1 week and 1 month after the conclusion of the treatment, for pain levels, measured using visual analogue scales (VAS) and an algometer (see Chapter 5).
- Range of motion of the neck was also tested.
- There was significant improvement in pain levels, and in the range of motion, in those people receiving magnetic treatment. The improvement was maintained up to and including a month after the treatment.
- The patients receiving placebo (dummy ultrasound) showed no benefit (Smania et al 2003).

Conclusion

Use of magnets and magnetic stimulation seems both safe and potentially effective.

Box 9.4   Metabolic and nutritional treatment

Simons et al (1999) reported that underactive thyroid function encourages and maintains myofascial trigger point activity.

They say that in some patients, the irritability of trigger points appears to be a clear indicator of just how low thyroid function is.

Unfortunately, when tested for thyroid hormone function many patients only show very mild underactivity, with thyroid hormone levels in blood samples being recorded as 'low normal', or 'borderline low'.

In such patients myofascial therapy may offer only temporary relief.

Experience suggests that the increased irritability of the muscles of such patients, and their failure to respond to physical treatment, improves when supplemental thyroid hormone, especially T3, is used.

In some patients there may be adequate thyroid hormone circulating, but there may be a cellular resistance to its activities, just as some people with diabetes have adequate insulin, which fails to 'work' as it should.

Treatment that adds thyroid hormone (desiccated thyroid or T3) in such cases is very controversial, and should only be undertaken by a practitioner who is licensed to do so, and who is fully trained in the use of endocrine products. Patients receiving thyroid hormone should be closely monitored.

Lowe (1997, 2000) and Lowe & Honeman Lowe (1998) make the guidelines clear, saying that it is essential to:

1. select the proper form of thyroid hormone
2. prepare the dosage properly
3. encourage patients to engage in activities or appropriate lifestyle changes.

Special precautions are taken with the elderly, and with people who are deconditioned, osteoporotic and/or have cardiac problems.

An example is given by Lowe as to where trigger points fit into treatment of fibromyalgia syndrome, when using thyroid hormone replacement (he calls the method *metabolic therapy*):

> Some patients who respond well to metabolic therapy, but who do not have physical treatment, are left with regional musculoskeletal pain they may misinterpret as persisting fibromyalgia.

He suggests that metabolic treatment prepares the tissues for more effective manual deactivation of trigger points in patients with widespread pain such as fibromyalgia who are also thyroid deficient.

Figure 9.3 shows a graph of pain in someone with fibromyalgia.

- There was a reduction in trigger point (and other) pain between weeks 1 and 5, while thyroid hormone was being taken.
- A plateau was reached between weeks 6 and 10, during which time almost no further pain reduction took place.
- Manual deactivation of trigger points started on week 10, after which pain levels dropped dramatically until, by week 15 there was hardly any pain at all.

Nutrition

A poor nutritional status, particularly if iron, vitamin C and the major B vitamins (folic acid, pyridoxine – B6, thiamine – B2 in particular) are deficient, seems to predispose toward, or aggravate, trigger point development and activity (Simons et al 1999).

Simons et al (1999) also reported that food allergies can aggravate trigger point activity. 'When the allergic symptoms are controlled the muscle response to local trigger point therapy usually improves significantly.'

So if someone has food allergies, this needs to be considered as an aggravating factor in maintaining the trigger point activity.

Simons et al also report on the aggravating influence of alcohol on trigger point activity, and the mixed effects of caffeine.

It seems that moderate amounts of caffeine may actually reduce trigger point activity by improving local circulation. But, 'excessive intake of coffee, and/or cola drinks that contain caffeine (more than 2 cups, bottles or cans daily), is likely to aggravate trigger point activity'.

Conclusion

Metabolic therapy (thyroid hormone replacement) seems to offer benefits to those people who display cellular resistance to normal levels of thyroid hormone in their bloodstream.

This form of treatment is potentially dangerous without supervision and close monitoring, and should be undertaken only by appropriately licensed, skilled and experienced practitioners.

Box 9.4   Metabolic and nutritional treatment – *cont'd*

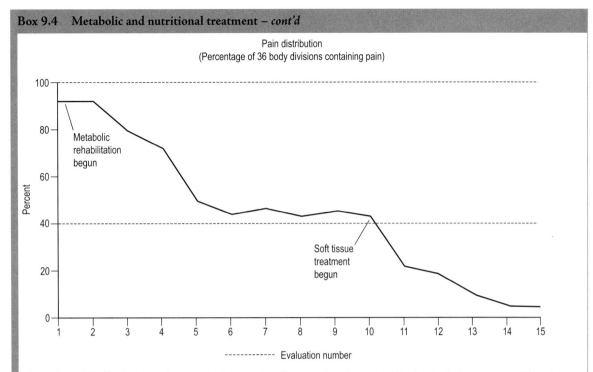

Figure 9.3   The line in the graph shows the decreases in a fibromyalgia patient's pain distribution during treatment. The pain distribution is the percentage of 36 body divisions containing pain, indicated by her on her pain drawing. Her pain distribution decreased during the first six weekly evaluations. The distribution did not decrease further until soft tissue treatment was begun, at the time of the tenth evaluation, to desensitize several myofascial trigger points. (Redrawn from *Journal of Bodywork and Movement Therapies* 4(1):211.)

Box 9.5   Microcurrent treatment

Microcurrent therapy uses extremely low currents (a millionth of an amp) that are passed through the nervous system via graphite gloves worn by the therapist (or wrapped in a damp towel and rested on the body) (Fig. 9.4).

Microcurrent has no relationship to TENS, which uses far higher currents in an attempt to mask pain sensations, and which shows very little value in treatment of trigger points.

The microcurrent produces no sensation at all (unlike TENS), and appears to mimic the natural physiological nerve transmissions (McMakin 1998).

Animal studies suggest that the effect is an enhancement of ATP (energy) production (Cheng 1982).

See Chapter 2 for an explanation of how low energy levels (ATP) seem to be a feature of trigger point activity, where its deficiency prevents, or delays, spontaneous recovery of the 'energy crisis' at the heart of the trigger point.

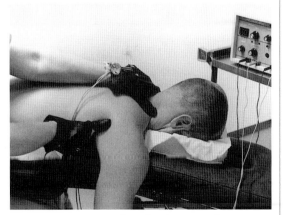

Figure 9.4   Prone cervical myofascial treatment focuses on the cervical paraspinals, the levator and trapezius, the serratus anterior and the subscapularis. (From Chaitow 2002.)

Box 9.5   Microcurrent treatment – *cont'd*

Microcurrent has been found to be very effective in treatment of pain of all sorts, and myofascial (trigger point) pain in particular (Kirsch 1997).

The updated text by Simons et al (1999) recommends microcurrent as a potentially valuable treatment method. McMakin (1998) reports that:

In 1996 we examined the results in 137 cases of 'simple' chronic myofascial pain, in various body regions, in patients who had no other musculoskeletal problem that might be causing the pain.

- Most of the conditions were due to trauma or chronic overuse.
- Symptoms had been present for from 8 months to 22 years.
- The majority of patients had previously been treated unsuccessfully by a range of methods, including prescription drugs, physical therapy, surgery, chiropractic, acupuncture, trigger point therapy and massage.
- Of the 137 patients, 128 completed treatment.
- Pain was reduced in 126 of those 128, from an average of between 5 and 8 out of 10, to 2 out of 10.
- Two patients had pain reduced from between 5 and 8 out of 10, to between 3 and 4 out of 10.
- Treatment duration varied depending on the severity, chronicity and complexity of each case, but most had significantly improved within 4 weeks.
- Random follow-up contacts suggest that the results have been long-lasting and possibly permanent.

Conclusion
Microcurrent seems to be both safe and effective as a treatment of myofascial pain.

Box 9.6   Ultrasound

There have been very few studies of the potential benefits of ultrasound treatment of trigger point pain.

One study evaluated treatment of trigger points in patients with neck and shoulder myofascial pain (Gam et al 1998).

- Some of the patients received ultrasound with home exercise and massage.
- Others received dummy ultrasound with home exercise and massage.
- Others had no treatment and acted as a control group.

- Both groups receiving treatment showed significant improvements in the number and sensitivity of trigger points. However, the ultrasound produced no additional advantage over and above the benefits of massage and exercise.

Conclusion
Although quite widely used in physiotherapy settings, there is no good evidence of usefulness of ultrasound in treating myofascial pain.

Box 9.7   Creams, ointments and essential oils

Capsaicin cream, which is available over-the-counter, stimulates local circulation and produces an erythema (redness). It contains chemicals that have a local pain-killing effect, and is thought to be particularly useful for treating trigger points close to scars.

If the cream is overused, however, the nerve cells that it influences become desensitized, and it will no longer work (Simons et al 1999).

Prescription only ointments, such as Quotane (dimethisoquin hydrochloride), have an anesthetic effect, and are recommended for use on superficial tissues, such as those on the face and head (McPartland 2004).

Starlanyl & Copeland (1996) recommend the use of a variety of essential oils that contain a compound called linalool, in treatment of trigger points. The oils can be rubbed onto the skin, as part of a massage, or used in bathing. The benefits deriving from the oils seem to be due to a reduction of the excessive release of acetylcholine, which is part of the trigger point mechanism (see Chapter 2 and Fig. 2.12).

Oils of particular value include: lavender, lemon balm, rosemary, passiflora, rose and valerian.

Conclusion
There appears to be very real benefit in terms of pain relief from these methods, although all would be short term unless the trigger points were deactivated.

Box 9.8   Hydrotherapy, balneotherapy and watsu

Methods used in traditional naturopathic practice to relieve musculoskeletal pain have a long history, as well as a great deal of personal testimony as to their value, but very little in the way of research validation (Boyle & Saine 1988).

Some of the methods described later in this section can be taught for home use. They should be presented to the patient as being of possible value, without certainty being implied.

The message that should be offered is something such as: 'These methods may help, but if they don't they can do no harm.'

Patients should be given a simple print-out with the details listed.

Evidence?
There is some research evidence of hydrotherapy being of value in controlled settings.

Hydrotherapy (particularly involving supervised exercises in sea water – balneotherapy) has been studied as a means of relieving general, body-wide, chronic pain as well as fibromyalgia pain (which almost always includes, as part of the total pain burden, myofascial trigger point pain).

Significant improvements have been observed in terms of reduced pain as well as enhanced function (Buskila et al 2001, Evcik et al 2002, Mannerkorpi et al 2000).

Sulfur baths and fibromyalgia syndrome (FMS)
Forty-eight patients with fibromyalgia were randomly assigned to a treatment group receiving sulfur baths, or a control group (Buskila et al 2001).

All participants stayed for 10 days at a Dead Sea spa.

Physical functioning, FMS-related symptoms and tenderness measurements (point count and pain threshold measurements) were assessed after 10 days of treatment, and 1 and 3 months after leaving the spa.

Relief in the severity of FMS-related symptoms (pain, fatigue, stiffness, and anxiety) and reduced frequency of symptoms (headache, sleep problems and subjective joint swelling) were reported in both groups, but lasted significantly longer in the treatment group.

Sleep enhancement via neutral bath
A 30 minute to 4 hour neutral bath (between 92°F/33.3°C and 97°F/36.1°C) has a calming influence and is also useful as a pain control method.

Indications
In all cases of anxiety, feelings of 'being stressed', and for relieving chronic pain and/or insomnia. To reduce serious fluid retention as in ascites, by means of hydrostatic pressure (Fawthrop et al 1987).

Method
- The bath should be run as full as possible, with the water as close to 97°F (36.1°C) as possible, and certainly *not* exceeding that level.
- Once in the bath, the water should cover the shoulders.
- A bath thermometer should be in the bath to ensure the temperature is maintained within a narrow range around 97°F/36.1°C.
- After the bath the person should rest.

Watsu
Watsu is a combination of massage (shia tsu) and movement in warm water (Dull 1997).

A New Zealand study (Faull 2005) looked at the effect of watsu on the pain being experienced by people with fibromyalgia (FMS):

> The results clearly indicate that Watsu has the potential to be an effective therapy that results in large health gains for people with FMS and therefore should be investigated further.

The researcher reported:

> Watsu claims to provide gains in physical, psychological, social and spiritual health. Watsu (WATer shiatSU) was developed in Northern California, during the early 1980s, by a Shiatsu practitioner who began to float people in warm water sourced from hot springs (35°C), while applying the moves and stretches of Zen Shiatsu. … The rhythmic movement through the water with accompanying massage are believed to facilitate relaxation, decrease pain, address abnormal muscle tone, muscle spasms as well as encourage deep breathing and relaxation.

Constitutional hydrotherapy – home application (Boyle & Saine 1988)
Constitutional hydrotherapy was developed by naturopaths in Washington State in the 1920s. It has a well-founded (but clinically unresearched) reputation as producing a non-specific 'balancing' effect, reducing chronic pain, enhancing immune function and promoting healing.

There are no contraindications since the degree of temperature contrast in its application can be modified to take account of any degree of sensitivity or frailty.

If the contrast between hot and cold is progressively increased, the results in terms of enhanced circulation, reduction in pain levels, and improved immune function are greater.

Box 9.8   Hydrotherapy, balneotherapy and watsu – *cont'd*

Ideally best results emerge over a 6- to 8-week period of almost daily application.

There is a need for someone to assist the person being treated, as it is impossible to apply constitutional hydrotherapy to yourself.

Method
1. Patient undresses and lies supine between sheets and under blanket.
2. Place two hot folded bath towels (four layers) onto patient's trunk, shoulders to hips, side to side.
3. Cover with sheet and blanket and leave for 5 minutes.
4. Return with a single layer (small) hot towel and a single layer cold towel.
5. Place 'new' hot towel onto top of four 'old' hot towels and 'flip' so that new hot towel is on skin and remove old towels.
6. Immediately place cold towel onto new hot towel and flip again so that cold is on the skin; remove single hot towel.
7. Cover patient with sheet and blanket, and leave for **10** minutes or until the cold towel is warmed.
8. Remove previously cold, now warm, towel and turn patient onto stomach.
9. Repeat steps 2 to 6 to the back of the patient.

Apply daily for weeks or months. The effect is to enhance immune function, reduce pain perception, and improve circulatory function.

Constitutional hydrotherapy: notes
1. If using a bed, take precautions not to get this wet.
2. 'Hot' water in this context is a temperature high enough to prevent you leaving your hand in it for more than 5 seconds.
3. The coldest water from a running tap is adequate for the 'cold' towel.
4. In hot summers adding ice to the water in which this towel is wrung out is acceptable, if the temperature contrast is acceptable to the patient.
5. If the patient feels cold after the cold towel is placed use back massage, foot or hand massage – through the blanket and towel) and/or use visualization – ask the patient to think of a sunny beach, for example.
6. Most importantly – by varying the differential between hot and cold, making it a small difference for someone whose immune function and overall degree of vulnerability is poor, for example, and using a large contrast, very hot and very cold, for someone whose constitution is robust, allows for the application of the method to anyone at all.
7. Apply daily or twice daily if needed.

Conclusion
There is good evidence of general health, and pain-relieving, (and sleep-enhancing), benefits from various forms of hydrotherapy.

CLINICAL NOTE

Key points from Chapter 9

1. There are mixed reports as to the value of needling techniques (acupuncture, dry needling, injections of medication), with dry needling being particularly likely to cause post-treatment tissue damage, making it less appropriate for sensitive and fragile patients.

2. Gentle needling (as described in Box 9.1) is, however, a suitable treatment for even very sensitive patients.

3. A variety of non-manual methods are being used to treat trigger points and widespread musculoskeletal pain, ranging from use of magnets, hydrotherapy and microcurrent (all safe and potentially beneficial), to ultrasound and laser treatment (no proven value) and metabolic therapy (potentially beneficial in appropriate cases, but with possible risks if not well supervised) as well as topical creams and oils (some short-term value).

References

Alvarez D J, Rockwell P G 2002 Trigger points: diagnosis and management. American Family Physician 65(4):653–660

Baldry P 1993 Acupuncture, trigger points and musculoskeletal pain. Churchill Livingstone, Edinburgh

Baldry P 2002 Acupuncture treatment of fibromyalgia and muscle pain. In: Chaitow L (ed) Fibromyalgia syndrome: a practitioner's guide to treatment. Churchill Livingstone, Edinburgh, p 113–127

Bowsher D 1990 Physiology and pathophysiology of pain. Journal of the British Medical Acupuncture Society 7:17–20

Boyle W, Saine A 1988 Naturopathic hydrotherapy. Buckeye Naturopathic Press, East Palestine, OH

Brown C, Parker N, Ling F et al 2000 Effect of magnets on chronic pelvic pain. Monday Posters 95(4):29S

Buskila D, Abu-Shakra M, Neumann L et al 2001 Balneotherapy for fibromyalgia at the Dead Sea. Rheumatology International 20(3):105–108

Chaitow L (ed) 2002 Fibromyalgia syndrome: a practitioner's guide to treatment. Churchill Livingstone, Edinburgh

Chaitow L 2003 Modern neuromuscular techniques, 2nd edn. Churchill Livingstone, Edinburgh

Cheng N 1982 The effect of electric currents on ATP generation, protein synthesis and membrane transport in rat skin. Clinical Orthopedics 171:264–272

Cheshire W, Abashian S, Mann J 1994 Botulinum toxin in the treatment of myofascial pain syndrome. Pain 59:65–69

Dull H 1997 Watsu: freeing the body in water, 2nd edn. Harbin Springs Publishing, Harbin, CA

Evcik D, Kizilay B, Gokcen E 2002 The effects of balneotherapy on fibromyalgia patients. Rheumatology International 22(2):56–59

Faull K 2005 Comparison of the effectiveness of watsu and Aix massage for those with fibromyalgia syndrome: a pilot study. Journal of Bodywork and Movement Therapies (in press)

Fawthrop F, O'Hare J P, Millar N et al 1987 Combined use of water immersion and frusemide in treatment of resistant ascites in liver cirrhosis. Journal of the Royal Society of Medicine 80(12):776–777

Frost F, Jessen B, Siggard-Andersen J 1980 A control, double blind comparison of mepivicaine injection versus saline injection for myofascial pain. Lancet 8167:499–500

Gam A, Warming S, Larsen L 1998. Treatment of myofascial trigger points with ultrasound combined with massage and exercise – a randomised controlled trial. Pain 77:73–79

Garvey T A, Marks M R, Wiesel S W 1989 A prospective, randomised, double blind evaluation of trigger point therapy for lower back pain. Spine 14:962–964

Gupta S, Schlifstein T, Varlotta G 2003 Improved clinical outcomes in trigger points injections by combined use of lidocaine, Toradol, and steroids. Poster 68. Archives of Physical Medicine and Rehabilitation Vol 84

Hameroff S R, Crago B R, Blitt C D et al 1981 Comparison of bupivacaine, etidocaine and saline for trigger point therapy. Anesthesia and Analgesia 60:752–755

Hong C-Z 1994 Considerations and recommendations regarding myofascial trigger points. Journal of Musculoskeletal Pain 2(1):29–59

Huguenin L 2004 Myofascial trigger points: the current evidence. Physical Therapy in Sport 5(1):2–12

Ingber R 2000 Shoulder impingement in tennis/racquetball players treated with subscapularis myofascial treatments. Archives of Physical Rehabilitation 181:679–682

Irnich D, Behrens N, Gleditsch J et al 2002 Immediate effects of dry needling and acupuncture at distant points in chronic neck pain: results of a randomised, double blind, sham-controlled crossover trial. Pain 99:83–89

Jones L 1981 Strain and counterstrain. Academy of Applied Osteopathy, Colorado Springs

Karakurum B, Karaalin O, Coskun O 2001 The dry needle technique: intramuscular stimulation in tension-type headache. Cephalalgia 21:813–817

Kawakita K, Itoh K, Okada K 2002 The polymodal receptor hypothesis of acupuncture and moxibustion, and its rational explanation of acupuncture points. International Congress Series: Acupuncture – is there a physiological basis? Elsevier Science, Amsterdam, 1238:63–68

Kirsch D 1997 How to achieve optimum results using microcurrent electrical therapy for pain management, part II. American Chiropractor (Sept/Oct):12–14

Lewit K 1979 The needle effect in the relief of myofascial pain. Pain 6:83–90

Lowe J C 1997 Thyroid status of 38 fibromyalgia patients: implications for the etiology of fibromyalgia. Clinical Bulletin of Myofascial Therapy 2(1):36–41

Lowe J C 2000 The metabolic treatment of fibromyalgia. McDowell Publishing Company, Boulder

Lowe J C, Honeyman-Lowe G 1998 Facilitating the decrease in fibromyalgic pain during metabolic rehabilitation: an essential role for soft tissue therapies. Journal of Bodywork and Movement Therapies 2(4):1–9

McMakin C 1998 Microcurrent treatment of myofascial pain in the head, neck and face. Topics in Clinical Chiropractic 5(1):29–35

McPartland J 2004 Travell trigger points – molecular and osteopathic perspectives. Journal of the American Osteopathic Association 104(6):244–249

Mann F 1963 The treatment of disease by acupuncture. Heinemann Medical, London

Mannerkorpi K, Nyberg B, Ahlmen M, Ekdahl C 2000 Pool exercise combined with an education program for patients with FMS. A prospective, randomized study. Journal of Rheumatology 27(1):2473–2481

Melzack R, Wall P 1989 Textbook of pain, 2nd edn. Churchill Livingstone, London

Melzack R, Stillwell D, Fox E 1977 Trigger points and acupuncture points for pain: correlations and implications. Pain 3:3–23

Olavi A, Pekka R, Pertii K 1989 Effects of the infrared laser therapy at treated and non-treated trigger points. Acupuncture and Electrotherapeutics Research 14(1):9–14

Simons D, Travell J, Simons L 1999 Myofascial pain and dysfunction: the trigger point manual. Vol 1: The upper body, 2nd edn. Williams & Wilkins, Baltimore

Smania N, Corato E, Fiaschi A 2003 Therapeutic effects of peripheral repetitive magnetic stimulation on myofascial pain syndrome. Clinical Neurophysiology 114(2):350–358

Starlanyl D, Copeland M 1996 Fibromyalgia and chronic muscle pain syndrome. New Harbinger Publications, Oakland, CA

Thorsen H, Gam A, Svensson B 1992 Low level laser therapy for myofascial pain in the neck and shoulder girdle. A double-blind, cross-over study. Scandinavian Journal of Rheumatology 21:139–141

Waylonis G, Wilke S, O'Toole D 1988 Chronic myofascial pain: management by low-output helium–neon laser therapy. Archives of Physical Medicine and Rehabilitation 69:1017–1020

Wheeler A, Goolkasian P, Gretz S 1998 A randomized, double blind, prospective pilot study of botulinum toxin injection for refractory, unilateral, cervicothoracic, paraspinal, myofascial pain syndrome. Spine 23:1662–1667

Glossary

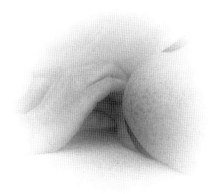

ah shi **points** Areas of local tenderness that do not have an obvious cause. In Traditional Chinese Medicine these are regarded as 'honorary' acupuncture points. *Ah shi* literally means 'ouch, it hurts'

Algometer A hand-held gauge used to measure how much pressure is being applied to a painful point

Anaerobic glycolysis The relatively inefficient production of energy by cells when there is a deficiency of oxygen. A process that produces acid wastes (lactic, pyruvic, etc)

Balneotherapy That part of hydrotherapy that describes the use of baths and their therapeutic use

Caudad Towards the feet, as compared to *cephalad* - towards the head (example : pressure was applied in a cephalad direction)

Cephalad Towards the head, as compared to *caudad* - towards the feet (example : pressure was applied in a caudad direction)

Decompensation When adaptation is exhausted, and dysfunction appears, tissues (joints, muscles, etc) will have become decompensated – for example in response to repetitive overuse

Dermatographia The appearance on the skin (derma) of marks in response to light pressure – literally being able to 'write on the skin'

Drag When used in the term 'drag palpation' this word refers to the light running of a finger or thumb tip across the skin to evaluate localized changes such as hydrosis (sweat) that signify sympathetic changes in underlying tissues. In those areas the finger tip fails to slide smoothly but 'drags'

Effleurage Used to describe the most basic form of rhythmic, gliding, massage stroke

Embryonic trigger point The earliest stage of a trigger point that develops in the 'target' tissues to which an active trigger point is referring sensations, such as pain

Energy production (ATP) Cells manufacture ATP (adenosine tri-phosphate), the raw material (chemical energy) that is released as mechanical energy. ATP fuels all bodily activities and functions and is stored in contractile tissues (e.g. muscle). A deficiency of ATP prevents trigger points from releasing the contracture at its heart

Enthesitis Dysfunction at the site of a muscle's attachment, involving inflammation, fibrosis and calcium deposition, which follows a process in those same tissues called enthesopathy, following – for example – repetitive stress of the tissues

Enthesopathy See previous definition

Facilitation The gradual sensitization (partial or sub-threshold excitation) of nerve tissues as a result of either mechanical stress, or reflex feedback to the tissues, from organ dysfunction. This can occur spinally (known as segmental facilitation) or locally (trigger point)

Fibromyalgia A condition defined by virtually constant, bodywide, pain and fatigue, commonly associated with a number of other symptoms including irritable bowel, poor sleep patterns and loss of short-term memory and concentration

Hydrotherapy The use of water (or ice or steam) therapeutically

Hyperalgesic skin zone (HSZ) A term coined by Karel Lewit MD to define localized areas of extreme skin sensitivity that commonly overlie trigger points and other facilitated (sensitized) areas – characterized by changes that can be palpated by 'drag palpation'

Magnetic coil stimulator Equipment that generates a magnetic field, used medically (for example) to 'jump-start' healing following bone fracture

Nociceptors Nerves that register pain

Parasympathetic nervous system The part of the autonomic nervous system that produces calm and relaxation, in contrast to the sympathetic nervous system that induces arousal (alarm response)

Petrissage Used to describe a wringing, pressing and stretching massage stroke that attempts to 'milk' the tissues of waste products and enhance circulation

Phasic muscles A muscle that has as its primary role the actions of movement, rather than maintenance of stability

Postural muscles A muscle that has as its primary role the actions of maintenance of stability rather than production of movement

Proprioceptors Nerve cells that report to the central nervous system and brain, information relating to (for example) the position and rate of movement of the tissues in which they lie

SAID (specific adaptation to imposed demand) The process of adaptation to specific activities – for example lifting weights, or running, which we commonly describe as 'training'

Satellite point A trigger point that evolves distant to an already active trigger point, which starts as an embryonic points (see above)

Somatovisceral A reflex that passes from the body tissues (soma) to an organ (viscera)

STAR palpation An acronym that identifies Sensitivity, Tenderness, Asymmetry and Range of motion changes

Sympathetic arousal A change that follows an alarm event, commonly thought of as the 'fight or flight' sensation

Sympathetic nervous system The part of the autonomic nervous system that produces arousal (see previous definition) in contrast to the parasympathetic nervous system

TENS Transcutaneous electrical nerve stimulation – a device used to ease pain

Type 1 fibers The predominant fiber type in postural muscles

Type 2 fibers The predominant fiber type in phasic muscles

Viscerosomatic A reflex that passes from an organ (viscera) to body tissues (soma)

Visual analogue scale This term usually applies to a line that is (say) 10 centimeters long, on which a mark is made to indicate the level of pain, or degree of distress being experienced of any symptom, where '0' represents no pain and '10' represents the worst pain imaginable.

Watsu Shiatsu applied with the patient and the therapist in a pool – a form of hydrotherapy.

Index

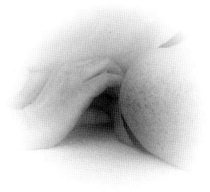

ELSEVIER DVD-ROM LICENCE AGREEMENT

PLEASE READ THE FOLLOWING AGREEMENT CAREFULLY BEFORE USING THIS PRODUCT. THIS PRODUCT IS LICENSED UNDER THE TERMS CONTAINED IN THIS LICENCE AGREEMENT ("Agreement"). BY USING THIS PRODUCT, YOU, AN INDIVIDUAL OR ENTITY INCLUDING EMPLOYEES, AGENTS AND REPRESENTATIVES ("You" or "Your"), ACKNOWLEDGE THAT YOU HAVE READ THIS AGREEMENT, THAT YOU UNDERSTAND IT, AND THAT YOU AGREE TO BE BOUND BY THE TERMS AND CONDITIONS OF THIS AGREEMENT. ELSEVIER LIMITED ("Elsevier") EXPRESSLY DOES NOT AGREE TO LICENSE THIS PRODUCT TO YOU UNLESS YOU ASSENT TO THIS AGREEMENT. IF YOU DO NOT AGREE WITH ANY OF THE FOLLOWING TERMS, YOU MAY, WITHIN THIRTY (30) DAYS AFTER YOUR RECEIPT OF THIS PRODUCT RETURN THE UNUSED PRODUCT AND ALL ACCOMPANYING DOCUMENTATION TO ELSEVIER FOR A FULL REFUND.

DEFINITIONS **As used in this Agreement, these terms shall have the following meanings:**

"Proprietary Material" means the valuable and proprietary information content of this Product including without limitation all indexes and graphic materials and software used to access, index, search and retrieve the information content from this Product developed or licensed by Elsevier and/or its affiliates, suppliers and licensors.

"Product" means the copy of the Proprietary Material and any other material delivered on DVD-ROM and any other human readable or machine-readable materials enclosed with this Agreement, including without limitation documentation relating to the same.

OWNERSHIP This Product has been supplied by and is proprietary to Elsevier and/or its affiliates, suppliers and licensors. The copyright in the Product belongs to Elsevier and/or its affiliates, suppliers and licensors and is protected by the copyright, trademark, trade secret and other intellectual property laws of the United Kingdom and international treaty provisions, including without limitation the Universal Copyright Convention and the Berne Copyright Convention. You have no ownership rights in this Product. Except as expressly set forth herein, no part of this Product, including without limitation the Proprietary Material, may be modified, copied or distributed in hardcopy or machine-readable form without prior written consent from Elsevier. All rights not expressly granted to You herein are expressly reserved. Any other use of this Product by any person or entity is strictly prohibited and a violation of this Agreement.

SCOPE OF RIGHTS LICENSED (PERMITTED USES) Elsevier is granting to You a limited, non-exclusive, non-transferable licence to use this Product in accordance with the terms of this Agreement. You may use or provide access to this Product on a single computer or terminal physically located at Your premises and in a secure network or move this Product to and use it on another single computer or terminal at the same location for personal use only, but under no circumstances may You

use or provide access to any part or parts of this Product on more than one computer or terminal simultaneously.

You shall not (a) copy, download, or otherwise reproduce the Product or any part(s) thereof in any medium, including, without limitation, online transmissions, local area networks, wide area networks, intranets, extranets and the Internet, or in any way, in whole or in part, except for printing out or downloading nonsubstantial portions of the text and images in the Product for Your own personal use; (b) alter, modify, or adapt the Product or any part(s) thereof, including but not limited to decompiling, disassembling, reverse engineering, or creating derivative works, without the prior written approval of Elsevier; (c) sell, license or otherwise distribute to third parties the Product or any part(s) thereof; or (d) alter, remove, obscure or obstruct the display of any copyright, trademark or other proprietary notice on or in the Product or on any printout or download of portions of the Proprietary Materials.

RESTRICTIONS ON TRANSFER This Licence is personal to You and neither Your rights hereunder nor the tangible embodiments of this Product, including without limitation the Proprietary Material, may be sold, assigned, transferred or sublicensed to any other person, including without limitation by operation of law, without the prior written consent of Elsevier. Any purported sale, assignment, transfer or sublicense without the prior written consent of Elsevier will be void and will automatically terminate the Licence granted hereunder.

TERM This Agreement will remain in effect until terminated pursuant to the terms of this Agreement. You may terminate this Agreement at any time by removing from Your system and destroying the Product and any copies of the Proprietary Material. Unauthorized copying of the Product, including without

limitation, the Proprietary Material and documentation, or otherwise failing to comply with the terms and conditions of this Agreement shall result in automatic termination of this licence and will make available to Elsevier legal remedies. Upon termination of this Agreement, the licence granted herein will terminate and You must immediately destroy the Product and all copies of the Product and of the Proprietary Material, together with any and all accompanying documentation. All provisions relating to proprietary rights shall survive termination of this Agreement.

LIMITED WARRANTY AND LIMITATION OF LIABILITY Elsevier warrants that the software embodied in this Product will perform in substantial compliance with the documentation supplied in this Product, unless the performance problems are the result of hardware failure or improper use. If You report a significant defect in performance in writing to Elsevier within ninety (90) calendar days of your having purchased the Product, and Elsevier is not able to correct same within sixty (60) days after its receipt of Your notification, You may return this Product, including all copies and documentation, to Elsevier and Elsevier will refund Your money. In order to apply for a refund on your purchased Product, please contact the return address on the invoice to obtain the refund request form ("Refund Request Form"), and either fax or mail your signed request and your proof of purchase to the address indicated on the Refund Request Form. Incomplete forms will not be processed. Defined terms in the Refund Request Form shall have the same meaning as in this Agreement.

YOU UNDERSTAND THAT, EXCEPT FOR THE LIMITED WARRANTY RECITED ABOVE, ELSEVIER, ITS AFFILIATES, LICENSORS, THIRD PARTY SUPPLIERS AND AGENTS (TOGETHER "THE SUPPLIERS") MAKE NO REPRESENTATIONS OR WARRANTIES, WITH RESPECT TO THE PRODUCT, INCLUDING, WITHOUT LIMITATION THE PROPRIETARY MATERIAL. ALL OTHER REPRESENTATIONS, WARRANTIES, CONDITIONS OR OTHER TERMS, WHETHER EXPRESS OR IMPLIED BY STATUTE OR COMMON LAW, ARE HEREBY EXCLUDED TO THE FULLEST EXTENT PERMITTED BY LAW.

IN PARTICULAR BUT WITHOUT LIMITATION TO THE FOREGOING NONE OF THE SUPPLIERS MAKE ANY REPRESENTATIONS OR WARRANTIES (WHETHER EXPRESS OR IMPLIED) REGARDING THE PERFORMANCE OF YOUR PAD, NETWORK OR COMPUTER SYSTEM WHEN USED IN CONJUNCTION WITH THE PRODUCT, NOR THAT THE PRODUCT WILL MEET YOUR REQUIREMENTS OR THAT ITS OPERATION WILL BE UNINTERRUPTED OR ERROR-FREE.

EXCEPT IN RESPECT OF DEATH OR PERSONAL INJURY CAUSED BY THE SUPPLIERS' NEGLIGENCE AND TO THE FULLEST EXTENT PERMITTED BY LAW, IN NO EVENT (AND REGARDLESS OF WHETHER SUCH DAMAGES ARE FORESEEABLE AND OF WHETHER SUCH LIABILITY IS BASED IN TORT, CONTRACT OR OTHERWISE) WILL ANY OF THE SUPPLIERS BE LIABLE TO YOU FOR ANY DAMAGES (INCLUDING, WITHOUT LIMITATION, ANY LOST PROFITS, LOST SAVINGS OR OTHER SPECIAL, INDIRECT, INCIDENTAL OR CONSEQUENTIAL DAMAGES ARISING OUT OF OR RESULTING FROM: (I) YOUR USE OF, OR INABILITY TO USE, THE PRODUCT; (II) DATA LOSS OR CORRUPTION; AND/OR (III) ERRORS OR OMISSIONS IN THE PROPRIETARY MATERIAL.

IF THE FOREGOING LIMITATION IS HELD TO BE UNENFORCEABLE, OUR MAXIMUM LIABILITY TO YOU IN RESPECT THEREOF SHALL NOT EXCEED THE AMOUNT OF THE LICENCE FEE PAID BY YOU FOR THE PRODUCT. THE REMEDIES AVAILABLE TO YOU AGAINST ELSEVIER AND THE LICENSORS OF MATERIALS INCLUDED IN THE PRODUCT ARE EXCLUSIVE.

If the information provided In the Product contains medical or health sciences information, it is intended for professional use within the medical field. Information about medical treatment or drug dosages is intended strictly for professional use, and because of rapid advances in the medical sciences, independent verification of diagnosis and drug dosages should be made. The provisions of this Agreement shall be severable, and in the event that any provision of this Agreement is found to be legally unenforceable, such unenforceability shall not prevent the enforcement or any other provision of this Agreement.

GOVERNING LAW This Agreement shall be governed by the laws of England and Wales. In any dispute arising out of this Agreement, you and Elsevier each consent to the exclusive personal jurisdiction and venue in the courts of England and Wales.

Minimum system requirements

Windows®
Windows 98 or higher
Pentium® processor-based PC
16 MB RAM (32 MB recommended)
10 MB of available hard-disk space
2 X or faster DVD-ROM drive
VGA monitor supporting thousands of colours (16-bit)

Macintosh®
Apple Power Macintosh
Mac OS version 9 or later
64 MB of available RAM
10 MB of available hard-disk space
2 X or faster DVD-ROM drive

NB: No data is transferred to the hard disk.
The DVD-ROM is self-contained and the application runs directly from the DVD-ROM.

Installation instructions

Windows®
If you have enabled DVD-ROM autoplay on your system then the DVD-ROM will run automatically when inserted into your DVD-ROM drive. If you have not enabled autoplay, click on My Computer and double-click on your DVD-Rom drive. Your DVD-ROM drive should be represented by an icon labeled 'Trigger'.

Macintosh®
If you have enabled DVD-ROM autoplay on your system then the DVD-ROM will run automatically when inserted into your DVD-ROM drive. If you have not enabled. Autoplay, click on the DVD-ROM icon that appears on your desktop, then click on 'Trigger' to open the application.

To enable the DVD-ROM to autorun, select the Control Panels from the Apple menu on your desktop. Select QuickTime settings, then select Autoplay. Click the Enable DVD-ROM Autoplay checkbox, and then save the settings.

Using this Product

Software Requirements
This product is designed to run with Internet Explorer 5.0 or later (PC) and Netscape 4.5 or later (Mac). Please refer to the help files on those programs for problems specific to the browser.

To use some of the functions on the DVD, the user must have the following:

a. DVD requires "Java Runtime Environment" to be installed in your system to use "Export" and "Slide Show" features. DVD automatically checks for "Java Runtime Environment" version 1.4.1 or later (PC) and MRJ 2.2.5 (Mac) if not available, it starts installing from the DVD. Please complete the installation process. Then click on the license agreement to proceed. "Java Runtime Environment" is available in the DVD's Software folder. If the user manually install the software, please make sure that the user start the application by clicking 'Trigger.exe'.
b. Your browser needs to be Java-enabled. If the user did not enable Java when installing your browser, the user may need to download some additional files from your browser manufacturer.
c. If your system does not support Autorun, then please explore the DVD contents, click on 'Trigger.exe' to start.
d. QuickTime version 6 or later must be installed in order to view the video clips. A version of QuickTime is available from www.apple.com/quicktime.

Acrobat Reader can be installed from the Software folder of the DVD.

Viewing Images
You can view images by chapter and export images to PowerPoint or an HTML presentation. Full details are available in the Help section of the DVD-Rom.

Technical Support
Technical support for this product is available between 7.30 a.m. and 7.00 p.m. CST, Monday through Friday. Before calling, be sure that your computer meets the minimum system requirements to run this software. Inside the United States and Canada, call 1-800-692-9010. Inside the United Kingdom, call 00-800-692-90100. Outside North America, call +1-314-872-8370. You may also fax your questions to +1-314-997-5080, or contact Technical Support through e-mail: technical.support@elsevier.com.